I0135667

HEALTH

How to Get, and How to Keep It

INTRODUCTION

The injunction "Know thyself" was inscribed in letters of gold over the portico of the temple of Delphi. We can know ourselves only by thoughtful observation and reflection. General forms of exercise may be presented, but we must consider whether our present health and physical condition will not require some modification of the prescribed forms. Certain modes of bathing and specific rules for diet and sleep may be good for the multitude and yet unsuited to particular individuals. Any marked change from our accustomed manner of life should begin gradually. For one who, in winter, has never taken any other than a warm or tepid bath, to plunge suddenly and without preparation into a tub of cold water might be attended with serious results, while by gradual stages the same point may be reached with positive advantage to health and comfort.

The popular error still prevails that a well equipped gymnasium and costly apparatus are necessary to healthful physical development. It is an important part of the object of this work to show that with little or no outlay for apparatus, and with the expenditure of very little time, both health and vigor may be secured and preserved, and the success and happiness of life be greatly promoted.

The hindrances to a more general adoption of a course of physical training as a means of promoting health and strength are:

1. Ignorance of the advantages to be secured.

2. Distrust of the efficiency of the methods.

3. Mistaken notions concerning cost of appliances.

4. The fear that too much time will be required to make the exercise profitable.

5. The belief that the old way is the best—to take your chances while you are well, and send for the doctor when you are ill.

The long lists of clergymen, comparatively young in years, but broken down in health, their usefulness gone, and themselves a burden upon the community, have taught the aspiring candidate for the ministry a useful lesson. The pulpit of to-day includes some of the most prominent college athletes, and all professional men acknowledge the benefits to be derived from physical training.

Who can fully estimate the value of health? It affects not only the happiness, but also the usefulness of every life. Without it, no substantial success can be achieved. By due attention to the simple laws of health, involving fresh air, pure water, wholesome food, sensible clothing, proper exercise, rest, and sleep, nine-tenths of all the ailments that afflict mankind, and the largest amount of human misery resulting therefrom, would be prevented.

AIR

Essentials of Life.—Air, water, and food are the great essentials of life. A man may go for days without food, and for hours without water, but deprive him of air, even for a few minutes, and he ceases to live. In quantity, the daily consumption of air far outmeasures the other two; in purity, it receives the least consideration. The city and the State alike exercise some oversight of the food and water supply of the people. Impurities in these often appeal to the sense of sight or smell or taste, and the individual is put on his guard. The intangible air is laden with the foulest and most poisonous substances, and is as freely inhaled as if it could make no difference to the health.

Lung Capacity.—The quantity of the air we breathe is also important. We may eat too much food, even though it be absolutely pure and wholesome, but we cannot consume too much pure air. The larger the lung space, therefore, the better for health and strength.

The full lung capacity of the average adult is about 330 cubic inches, but an ordinary inspiration does not take in more than one-eleventh part of that volume. The value of full, deep breathing, and of large lung capacity becomes at once apparent. The larger the quantity of air consumed, the greater the amount of life-giving oxygen conveyed through the blood to all parts of the body. No form of physical exercise, therefore, can exceed in value the breathing exercises described in another chapter.

Rate of Breathing.—It is estimated that we breathe once during every four beats of the heart, or about eighteen times a minute. The relation between the heart and lungs is so close that whatever modifies the pulse affects the breathing. When the heart action is hurried, more blood is sent to the lungs, requiring more rapid action on their part. About every fifth breath the inspiration is longer and fuller, the effect being to change more completely the air of the lungs.

Holding the Breath.—While respiration is, for the most part, involuntary, we may arrest the breathing for the space of twenty to thirty seconds. If we first fortify the lungs by taking several deep inspirations and expelling the impure air as fully as possible, we may hold the breath for a minute or two. This power will prove of advantage if we have occasion to pass through a room or hallway filled with smoke, or to remain under water for a brief time. The pearl-fishers, as a result of training, remain under water from three to four minutes.

Importance of Pure Air.—Pure air means pure blood. The air of the mountain tops or by the sea fills us with life, while that of narrow streets, crowded rooms, unventilated dwellings, schools, churches, and theatres is depressing, weakening, and death-dealing.

So far from the aristocracy having a monopoly of blue blood, it flows through the veins of high and low alike. It goes out from the lungs bright and rich with oxygen; it comes back to the heart dark with the waste and poisonous matters which it has gathered in its course.

Atmospheric air is composed of several gases, the principal elements being oxygen, nitrogen, and watery vapor. All animal life requires oxygen for the combustion of the material supplied through the blood. The blood makes its circuit through the body three times a minute. It comes to the lungs laden with poisonous matter. Nearly one-third of the excretions of the body are eliminated through the lungs. The average adult contaminates about five thousand cubic inches of air with every breath. The importance of having an abundant supply of pure air at all times is obvious.

In ordinary respiration an adult abstracts sixteen cubic feet of oxygen from the atmosphere every twenty-four hours, and adds to it fourteen cubic feet of carbonic acid in the same time. If the individual were confined in a close apartment, in which the air could not mingle with the atmosphere without, the processes of life could not long be maintained.

History furnishes many instances of the direful effects of crowding a number of human beings into a limited space without ventilation. One hundred and fifty passengers were confined in the small cabin of a steamship one stormy night, and when morning came only eighty were found alive. Three hundred prisoners, after the battle of Austerlitz, were crowded into a close prison, and within a few hours two hundred and sixty of them had died.

The effects of foul air are not usually so sudden nor so striking. More frequently they consist of a general deficiency of nutrition, loss of vigor of body and mind, and of the power of resistance to disease. Consumptive patients, in a large majority of cases, come from the classes whose occupations confine them to ill-ventilated rooms. A cramped position of the body while at work, and want of good wholesome food, contribute to the mortality from this cause.

Absolutely pure air is rarely found in nature. Even in the open country there are three parts of carbonic acid in ten thousand parts of air. In cities and towns, the out-door air contains from four to five parts of carbonic acid. When, in dwellings and churches and halls, it reaches six to seven parts, its impurity is detected by the nose, the lungs suffer from a lack of oxygen, and the room feels close and stuffy.

The amount of carbonic acid in the breath is about five per cent. Air once used is therefore unfit for purposes of animal combustion. If breathed into a jar containing a short lighted candle, it will at once extinguish the flame. It would also prove fatal to small birds or mice. When the carbonic acid reaches one part in ten of common air, it becomes fatal to man.

Headaches, dullness, drowsiness, and labored respiration are the first symptoms of this lung poison. Faintness, convulsions, and unconsciousness are a later stage. School-houses, churches, theatres, and factories should be so well ventilated that the proportion of carbonic acid would not exceed two parts in one thousand.

Effects of Breathing Impure Air.—Air which is only slightly vitiated, if breathed day after day, for a considerable time, produces most serious results. Its effects are seen in pale faces, loss of appetite, depressed spirits, and a lack of muscular vigor.

An investigation made some years ago showed 86 deaths per 1,000 in a badly ventilated prison, and of these, 51.4 per 1,000 were due to phthisis, or consumption. In the House of Correction, in the same city, which was well ventilated, the death rate was 14 per 1,000, and of these only 7.9 were occasioned by phthisis. The organic particles thrown off from the lungs of diseased persons are responsible for the prevalence of phthisis and other lung diseases. It is also a well established fact that a bad atmosphere promotes the rapid spread of such specific diseases as small-pox, typhus, and scarlet fever.

Constant Supply.—Of so great importance is the matter of having a constant supply of unvitiated air that sanitariums for consumptives are now becoming common in which the principal feature is to have the patients enjoy a continuous out-door existence, day and night, being wrapped up and otherwise protected from cold and dampness. Consumptive symptoms often yield to this treatment.

Individual Habit.—Habit has much to do with our appreciation of pure air. If we recognize its value to health and to all the mental and physical activities, and insist upon a plentiful supply of pure oxygen, the habit soon becomes a second nature, and we instinctively feel uncomfortable upon entering an ill-ventilated room. In northern climates, economic considerations often interfere with the highest sanitary regulations. Householders, school boards, and church trustees frequently save fuel at the expense of health.

We may, however, by spending much time in poorly ventilated rooms, become so accustomed to the depressing influence of the impoverished atmosphere that we suffer a sort of semi-stupor without being conscious of the fact. How great a wrong is inflicted upon children in the school-room and in the crowded factory, by subjecting them, day after day, for months and years, to a vitiated atmosphere, laden with the poisonous exhalations from lungs and skin! Their growing bodies are stunted and their awakening intellects dulled, and the seeds of disease and weakness are implanted to develop into a harvest of wretchedness and misery in later life.

Sea Air.—When the breeze is off the ocean, the air is practically free from the exhalations of animals, the smoke and soot of chimneys, and the gases of sewers. The curative value of sea-air is well known. It comes richly laden with ozone, and its effect upon sojourners at the sea-side is very stimulating. Many persons are not strong enough to endure sea-bathing, yet gain much benefit from the sea-air.

Mountain Air.—The air of the mountains is pure. It is usually still, and seldom foggy. Being more rarefied than that of the low-lying valleys, it contains less oxygen in proportion to volume, but its lesser density gives to the oxygen greater activity.

The body loses heat less rapidly in rarefied atmospheres, so that there is probably less need of heat-production on the mountain than on the plain, combustion being less active. The rapid and great variations of temperature of the mountain regions stimulate the vital processes and contribute to the curative agencies of those altitudes.

Night Air.—There is a prevailing prejudice against night air. By many persons out-door air is shut out of the sleeping room as if it were pestilential. Analysis as well as experience shows that the most vitiated and unwholesome night air is that which has been breathed over and over again in a close sleeping apartment. Admit the outside air freely if you desire health. Guard against draughts, and use just enough bed covering for comfort.

Air of the School-Room.—A plentiful supply of pure air is desirable wherever there are people to breathe it. In no place is it more important than in the school-room. Confined for six hours each day during the period of life when the best health conditions are required for the proper growth of mind and body, the child thus robbed of the needed oxygen is wronged. The adult who voluntarily subjects himself once or twice a week for two hours to the poisonous atmosphere of church, lecture hall, or theatre, may experience a temporary headache, but is soon revived after reaching the fresh air. The child, ignorant of the wrong he is made to suffer, and incapable of providing better conditions, breathes the poisonous exhalations from fifty pairs of lungs, day after day, and thus has sown in his system the seeds of disease.

Illuminating Gas.—Many persons die every year by inhaling illuminating gas. People unacquainted with the use of gas fixtures often blow out the light instead of turning the key. A prevailing custom in some families is to keep the light burning low during the night. A variation of pressure in the pipes, or a sudden draught of air, extinguishes the slender flame, and gas escapes into the room, often with fatal results.

Leaky pipes or faulty fixtures may have the same effect. If the key be loose, tighten the screw that holds it in place. If there is a leak in the pipe or joint, which may be determined by applying a match, a gas-fitter should at once be summoned. Delay is dangerous and may prove fatal.

If a room be heavily charged with gas, get the windows and doors open as soon as possible. Do not go near with a light, lest an explosion follow. Naphtha and benzine are also highly explosive. When either is used to clean clothing, the work should be done in the open air, and never where the fumes may come in contact with the fire of stove or range, or with the flame of candle or lamp.

Gas burners, oil lamps, sperm candles, all forms of illuminants, consume the oxygen of a room and increase the carbonic acid. An oil lamp of ordinary dimensions gives off as much carbonic acid as an adult person. A man, seated in a room of moderate dimensions and using a good oil lamp, will require 6,000 cubic feet of fresh air every hour in order to keep the air from becoming vitiated beyond the point of wholesomeness. Gas from coal, coke, or charcoal fires is as dangerous as illuminating gas.

Heaters, ranges, stoves, and furnaces should be kept in complete order, so that no gas shall escape. Its entrance into a bedroom is often so stealthy as to stupefy the unconscious sleeper and destroy life without awakening him.

Sewer Gas.—Of all forms of vitiated air in cities, none is responsible for such serious derangement of health as that which is polluted by the air or gas from sewers and waste pipes. Some physicians and sanitarians hold that sewer air is often the direct cause of typhoid fever, scarlet fever, diphtheria, and cholera. Others maintain that the sewers and pipes furnish favorable breeding places for the germs of these diseases, which germs are carried through the air and produce their effects. The important matter is to keep the waste pipes flushed and well trapped. Some precautions against sewer gas are treated in the chapter on Dwellings.

Influence of Climate and Temperature.—Diarrhœal diseases, both of adults and children, are most frequent during hot weather. In July, August, and September there are from ten to twelve times as many cases as at other seasons of the year. Proper diet and suitable clothing will go far toward protecting the individual from the ill effects of climate and season.

The mortality from consumption and other forms of lung diseases is greatest in March and April, and least in August and September. September and October claim the greatest number of deaths from typhoid fever, followed closely by August and November. The mortality from diphtheria and croup is highest in November and December, and lowest in August and September. Of suicides, the largest number occur in May, and the fewest in February.

Hygienic Value of Winds.—Prof. Dexter, of the University of Illinois, has made a careful study of the effects of calms on the records of the public schools, the police courts, and the penitentiaries. All air movements not exceeding four miles an hour are regarded as calms. Over 497,000 observations were considered and tabulated. These show that during calm weather the absence from school on account of illness is three times as great as that during all other kinds of weather, including the very cold, wet, and windy. During calms, the criminal records show less disorder and violence, more policemen are laid off, more errors are made by clerks in banks, and more deaths are reported. This is in accordance with the principle that oxygen is the great source of mental and physical energy. When oxygen is deficient, we are less capable of action, either for good or evil. The slowly-moving air-currents of a large city are robbed of their oxygen, and vitiated by the exhalations of thousands of men and animals. A brisk wind brings in a fresh supply of vitalized air to take the place of the old, and to promote physical and mental energy. Old Boreas is a better friend than we have been wont to believe.

Nature's Balance.—By a wise provision of nature, the carbonic acid, which is so destructive to all animal life, constitutes the chief food of plants. These absorb the carbon and give out oxygen, and in this way the animal and vegetable kingdoms tend to preserve the balance of nature. Except for this wonderful provision, the human family would be threatened with annihilation.

WATER

Water in the Human Body.—Taken as a whole, the human body consists of about seventy-one parts of water in the hundred. When we consider how large a quantity of water is given off daily, not only through the kidneys and intestines, but through perspiration, sensible and insensible, and through the vapor breathed out from the lungs, it becomes clear that the food must contain a large proportion of water to supply the daily loss.

The proportions of water are not always quite the same, nor does the identical water present in any part of the body at any given moment remain there. There is a constant movement, a continual renewal going on in the body, and water helps to accomplish this renewal. By means of the watery substances, the saliva, the bile, and other juices of the stomach and intestines, the solid nutritive parts of the food are dissolved, and pass into the blood to renew the waste, and to keep up that continual current called life. Water is also useful in carrying off the worn out and useless materials which pass out through the fluid excretions and through the vapors from the lungs and skin.

Water in Food.—The amount of water contained in many articles of food that appear quite solid is generally surprising to those unacquainted with the chemistry of foods. In one hundred pounds by weight, fresh oatmeal contains 5 pounds of water. Corn and barley meal, wheat flour, peas, and beans contain 14 pounds; rice 15; bread 40; potatoes 75; grapes 80; parsnips 81; beets 82; apples 83; carrots and cabbages 89; onions 91; lettuce 96.

Of the animal foods, butter contains 10 pounds of water in one hundred; bacon 22; cheese 34; eggs 72; lean meat 73; fish 74; milk 86. By cooking, most foods lose a part of their natural moisture. The eatable part of a mutton chop contains 70 per cent of water before cooking, and 54 per cent after.

Daily Requirement.—Scientific sanitarians have estimated the daily requirement of water for a person at from twelve to sixteen gallons. The

British War Department aims to provide each soldier with fifteen gallons daily. In cities the daily allowance per capita is fifty gallons and upwards, which provides for animals, manufacturing purposes, fires, sewerage, etc., as well as for drinking, cooking, bathing, and other wants of man.

Sources of Supply.—The importance of an abundant supply of pure water is becoming more and more apparent each year. The numerous and serious epidemics throughout the country whose sources have been traced to the use of impure water leave no room for question on this point. Most cities draw their supplies from rivers and lakes. If these sources are kept free from sewage and the waste of manufacturing establishments the water is likely to be pure and wholesome. Subsiding reservoirs and filtration beds are needed to take out the mud occasioned by rains, and to catch up whatever floating matter may be carried into the basins. Muddiness is not always an indication of unwholesomeness, nor is clearness a proof of purity. Germs of disease have been found in the clearest water. Whenever there is the least suspicion of unwholesomeness, all water used for cooking and drinking should be boiled. It is not safe to trust to the theory, held by some, that a running stream, even if polluted, will in flowing a distance of twelve or fifteen miles purify itself.

Wells, which are the chief source of supply in the country, should be kept away from barnyards, stables, cesspools, and the waste waters from dairy and kitchen, to preserve them from pollution. Many cases of typhoid fever and other serious diseases have been directly traced to a violation of this rule. The ground surrounding the well should be raised so as to throw all surface water twelve or fifteen feet away from the well. See also what is said on this subject in the chapter on Dwellings.

Springs usually furnish the purest and best water. Coming from a considerable depth, spring-water loses, in its passage through the earth, most if not all its organic matter, and rises to the surface clear, cool, pure, and sparkling. The spring should be walled and covered, and otherwise protected from surface drainage.

Cisterns.—Rain-water collected in the country, and under favorable conditions, is comparatively pure and wholesome. In the cities, it contains such a large amount of organic matter and other impurities, washed out of the air and off the roofs by the rain and snow, that it is generally unfit for drinking without being filtered. On account of its softness, rain-water is very desirable for washing and other domestic purposes, but owing to the absence of mineral constituents it is flat and insipid to the taste. In New Orleans and other southern cities, where cisterns are largely used, the water is rendered cool and palatable by the use of large quantities of artificial ice.

Ice.—It was formerly supposed that in the process of freezing all deleterious matter contained in the water was excluded. Several outbreaks of disease in New England led to an investigation, which showed that the ice used had been taken from ponds whose waters contained large quantities of sewage and other impurities. A change in the source of the ice supply resulted in an immediate check of the disease. Recent research has shown that typhoid bacilli, after being frozen in a block of ice for 103 days, may still be alive when released.

Diseases Caused by Drinking Polluted Water.—A polluted water supply affects not one, but usually many persons, and notable epidemics have resulted. In consequence, more diligent inquiry has been instituted by Municipal, State, and National Boards of Health, and the evidence adduced is of the most positive character. Typhoid fever, cholera, dysentery, and diarrhœa have been clearly traced to the use of impure drinking water, and other related diseases are suspected of having a similar origin, although the evidence is not so conclusive.

Appearance.—A drinking water should be clear and bright. When shaken in a glass or bottle, bubbles should rise quickly and break immediately. If the bubbles move slowly, or seem to hang for some time in the water, they are probably due to the presence of decaying organic matter, and the water is of questionable purity. A slight cloudiness in the appearance of the water, following a rain, may be due to the presence of a small quantity of earthy matter, and not seriously affect its wholesomeness, but if the discoloration looks like that occasioned by a drop of milk the water should be avoided until carefully tested.

Smell.—A good water should have no smell. To this end, the cisterns or other receptacles must be kept perfectly clean. The purest and best waters will soon become foul if stored in unclean vessels.

Taste.—Water having a disagreeable taste is apt to be unwholesome. In order that we may derive from it proper nourishment, water, like other parts of our food, should be pleasant to the taste. And yet, the taste is by no means a satisfactory test of purity. The purest of all water is distilled water, which, by reason of the absence of all mineral matter and air, has a flat and insipid taste. The cleanest rain-water is also insipid. Boiled water is not much better, for while the boiling process may have destroyed all poisonous or noxious germs, and rendered the water absolutely wholesome, it also drove off the natural gases which gave to the water a pleasant taste. Boiled water may be re-aerated by pouring from an ordinary sprinkling can several times.

Hard Water.—Hardness is a serious drawback, whether the water be used for cooking, bathing, or for washing clothes. Food cooked by boiling in hard water is, as a rule, not so well prepared. Greens take on a gray color. Tea is never so good made from hard water. For cleaning the skin, hard water is not nearly so efficient as soft. Linens are never of a good color when washed in hard water.

Boiling hard water before using it improves it. A pinch or two of carbonate of soda, or of borax, is helpful in washing. A little table salt improves it for cooking most vegetables.

Filtration.—The following is a simple home-made filter. Take a large flower-pot, and soak it thoroughly in clean water. Stop up the hole in the bottom with a cork, in which insert a glass tube about three or four inches long. The top of the cork and tube should be nearly flat with the inside bottom of the pot. Put in a layer of sharp, clean sand about two inches deep, then two inches of small gravel, and three inches of well-burnt animal charcoal. On the top of this another layer of sand, and then another layer of gravel. The gravel, sand, and charcoal should be thoroughly washed before using. If the flow of water is too rapid, it may be checked by laying several flat pieces of glass upon the layers of sand. At reasonable intervals, the sand, gravel, and charcoal must be taken out, washed thoroughly, heated in the oven, and replaced in the pot, which must also be soaked in boiling water. This filter will remove nearly or quite all of the inorganic matter held in suspension in the water, but it is not to be depended upon to remove dangerous microbes and other germs of disease. If the water be thoroughly boiled for half an hour and cooled before being filtered, all danger will be removed.

There are many inexpensive filters on the market. They all become clogged, in a little while, and need to be cleaned or renewed. The cleaning of the one described above is so simple that any housekeeper could do it satisfactorily.

FOOD AND DRINK

Why We Eat.—During the early period of life, and until we reach maturity, food is necessary not only to repair the daily waste, but for the nurture and growth of the body. The intense bodily activity of childhood is attended with a large consumption of material and a great amount of waste. The food is converted into blood, which circulates through the arteries of the body, carrying the nutritive particles to the remotest parts, and returns through the veins, conveying the waste and worn out matter to be expelled from the system.

Quantity of Food.—Placing the average weight of an adult man at one hundred and forty-four pounds, the average daily amount of food and drink needed would be six pounds, or about one-twenty-fourth the weight of his body. Food should be taken in sufficient quantity to repair the waste, and no more. Most persons habitually eat and drink more than they need, while a few eat less than they should. Those who lead very active lives, or live much in the open air, require more food than the old, the inactive, and the sedentary. Habit, too, has much to do with the quantity of food taken. Over-indulgence in eating is the fruitful cause of a long train of evils. The appetite is pampered by tempting viands, and the stomach is overtaxed with work. The sensation of hunger is Nature's demand for food; the lack of such sensation should suggest abstinence.

Mixed Diet.—In infancy the digestive powers are weak and undeveloped, and food must be taken in its simplest form. Milk alone, at this period of life, seems best adapted to sustain life and growth. After this period has been passed, no single article of food furnishes all the principles necessary to support the growth, repair the waste, sustain the strength, and preserve the health. A mixed diet, therefore, becomes necessary.

Feeding Children.—There is no greater error in the management of children than that of giving them animal diet too early. That portion of the digestive apparatus intended to dispose of this kind of diet is in an embryonic condition up to a certain age, and in the efforts of digestion, inflammation, possibly convulsions and death, may follow as the immediate result.

Impaired digestion acquired in childhood is apt to continue through life. The structure of the human body being so largely dependent upon good, wholesome food taken at proper intervals, the importance of laying a good foundation in childhood needs no argument.

The practice of allowing children to eat at short intervals through the day is exceedingly deleterious. Cakes, nuts, fruit and other good things, in carefully regulated quantities, should form a part of the regular meal, when the children are old enough to have them, and should not be eaten between meals. When it is remembered that one-half of all the children born into the world die before reaching the age of sixteen, the importance of children's diet becomes apparent.

Selection.—In the selection of food, reference should be had to climate, season, occupation, and suitability. The races of the far North subsist largely on the blubber of seals and other fatty substances. In the winter season, persons living in the temperate zones require more of the heat-producing foods, and in summer, fruits and vegetables are more largely used. The man who leads an active out-door life consumes more oxygen, and requires not only more food, but of a kind that will rapidly build up muscle and impart strength. And not the least consideration, in the selection of food, is that of suitability or adaptation to the individual's condition or peculiarity. "What is one man's meat is another man's poison," says the old proverb. Most persons have found that certain fruits or vegetables or other articles of diet, which are generally considered wholesome, do not agree with them. It is important that each individual should study his peculiarities, in this respect, and abstain from eating or drinking those things which experience has shown will produce discomfort.

Happy is the man whose digestion is so perfect that he is never reminded that he has a stomach. But even those who cannot boast of such enviable powers of digestion, may yet, by a proper amount of exercise and the regulation of their diet, build up health and strength, and lead lives of usefulness and happiness, free from the many ills growing out of improper eating.

Proper Food.—Life is conditioned upon the proper supply of food. Men may, and do, exist upon very unsuitable food. To be able to do a good day's work within the hours of a reasonable working day is every man's birthright. Many men, like Esau of old, sell their birthright for a mess of pottage. Unlike him, however, they are not pressed by stress of hunger, but, merely to please the palate for five minutes, they burden the digestive organs for five hours, and repeat the process day after day. The comparison, therefore, is rather complimentary to Esau.

Constituents of the Body.—As already remarked, a large part of the human body is water. The body of a man weighing one hundred and fifty pounds contains less than fifty pounds of solid matter. The blood, brain, and nerves are about eighty per cent water; the muscles, nearly eighty per cent; and even the bones and the teeth contain a large percentage of water. Man may be deprived of solid food for a day or more without suffering, and, in some instances, persons have subsisted for several weeks on water alone, but to be deprived of water for ten or twelve hours causes much suffering.

The animal and vegetable kingdoms supply the organic substances which constitute a large part of the material commonly known as food, and which sustain the body in life and strength.

In addition, various inorganic substances enter into the human structure, prominent among which are salt, lime and iron. Salt is so important to animal life that herds of wild animals have been known to travel many miles to the salt-licks, or springs, in search of it. Some persons, from habit, use it to excess in seasoning their food. Lime and iron are taken into the body through the food. Iron forms about one part in a thousand of human blood.

Classification of Foods.—For increasing weight and producing heat, the fatty portions of meat, butter, and lard, together with wheat, Indian corn, and sugar, are best adapted; for muscle-making, lean meat, peas, beans, oatmeal; for brain and nerves, shell-fish, lean meats, peas, and beans. Those who lead an active, bustling life, especially if they take an abundance of out-door exercise, will naturally crave strong food in unstinted supply. The busy brain-worker, who is housed all day, and scarcely rises from his chair, needs to be much more careful in his diet. Coarse bread, lean meats, and fruits should constitute his chief dependence, with very limited use of butter, oils, and sugar.

Proper digestion depends upon the power of appropriating the food supplied, and this, in turn, upon the needs of the system. The best of food cannot be properly digested when it is not needed. All that the system requires will be used, and the rest will be cast out by the organs of excretion, which are often overtaxed, and the vital forces wasted, in the effort. The liver especially is burdened in its effort to carry off the excess of carbonaceous matter from the blood, and biliousness is the result. On the approach of warm weather, when the air has less oxygen to consume the food, this is particularly true.

Quantity.—We should eat to live, not live to eat. More people suffer from over-eating than from eating too little. Many thin people are large eaters, and stout people are often small eaters. The young generally eat more than the old. Not only are their powers of digestion better, due in part to the great amount of exercise they take, but they need food for growth, as well as to repair the waste. Franklin's prudent rule was to leave off eating with a good appetite.

Economy of the life forces requires that each person should strive to find out just how much food he requires to support his strength and repair the waste. One ounce more than is required is a triple waste,—a waste in the original cost, a waste of muscular force in digesting it, and a waste of nerve and vital force in getting rid of it.

Cereals and Their Food Value.—Dr. H. W. Wiley, Chief of the Bureau of Chemistry in the United States Department of Agriculture, in speaking of the substitutes for meat, says: "In so far as actual nourishment is concerned, the very cheapest and best that can be secured is presented by the cereals, viz., Indian corn, wheat, oats, rye, rice, etc. These contain all the nourishment necessary to supply the waste of the body and the energy and heat necessary to all animal functions and hard labor, in a form well suited to digestion, and capable not only of maintaining the body in a perfect condition, but also of furnishing the energy necessary to the hardest kind of manual labor. The waste material in cereals is very small, and, as compared with that in meats, practically none at all. In fact, the ordinary wastes, such as the bran and germ, are among the most nutritive components of the cereals, and both health and economy would be conserved, as a rule, by their consumption, instead of rejecting them as in the ordinary process of milling. The ordinary cereals of commerce contain only about ten per cent of waste, and this is an exceedingly small proportion, as compared with the percentage in meats.

"If meats should be used more for condimental purposes, as in the making of soups, stews, etc., and not more than once a day, as one of the staple articles of the table, it would be better, in my opinion, for the health and strength of the consumer, and especially would it be a saving in the matter of household expenses.

"It is well known that men who are nourished very extensively on cereals are capable of the hardest and most enduring manual labor. Meats are quickly digested, furnish an abundance of energy soon after consumption, but are not retained in the digestive organism long enough to sustain permanent muscular exertion. On the other hand, cereal foods are more slowly digested, furnish the energy necessary to digestion and the vital functions in a more uniform manner, and thus are better suited to sustain hard manual labor for a long period of time.

"The cereals contain all the elements necessary to the nutrition of the body, having in themselves the types of food which are represented by the fats, the nitrogenous or protein bodies, and the carbohydrates. In addition to these, they contain those mineral elements of which the bony structure of the body is composed, viz., lime and phosphoric acid. If, therefore, man were confined to a single article of diet, there is nothing which would be so suitable for his use as the cereals. Starch and sugar are primarily the foods which furnish animal heat and energy, and hence should be used in great abundance by those who are engaged in manual labor. The workingmen of our country, especially, should consider this point, and accustom themselves more and more to the use of cereals in their foods. When properly prepared and properly served they are palatable, as well as nutritious, and their judicious use in this way would tend to diminish the craving for flesh, which, however, it is not advisable to exclude entirely from the diet. By persons whose habits of life are sedentary, requiring but little physical exertion, starch and sugar should be eaten more sparingly."

Preparation of Foods.—No country equals our own in the abundance and quality of materials for the table, and probably no other compares with it in the ignorance and carelessness displayed in its cooking. A large part of the sickness, discomfort, and unhappiness of life finds its source just here. In many well-to-do families the whole matter is relegated to ignorant and incompetent servants whose only interest in the household is of a financial character, and that is entirely one-sided. The mistress is often more ignorant on this subject than the servant, and the "queen of the kitchen" reigns supreme.

Among the middle and lower classes, where the mistress is herself the cook, the results are no better. Being without proper early training, or growing up with the idea that it is not genteel to work, she comes to her task wholly unprepared, and an ill-fed, sickly family is the result. In many cities and towns, cooking schools are found, but the graduates do not compare with those who graduated from their mothers' kitchens, in the days when domestic labor was respected. The mind of the ambitious cooking-school graduate is too often concerned with the pretty pastries and dainty desserts that please the eye and pamper the appetite, instead of mastering the art of properly preparing the bread, meat, and vegetables, and the other substantial things.

Bread.—So important a part does bread play in the physical economy that it is often called the staff of life. In cities and towns and in many country villages the baker supplies the general need. Yielding to the popular demand for white bread, he uses flour that has been robbed of its most nutritious properties, and introduces unwholesome substances to make it light and white. The best bread is that in which the starch cells are most completely burst. The making of wholesome, palatable, home-made bread is becoming a "lost art" even among farmers' wives and daughters. The corner grocery and the baker's wagon furnish the freshly-baked loaf, the housewife is spared some trouble, and the household loses what should be one of the most healthful, nutritious, and appetizing elements of the daily supply of food. In parts of the South and West, the large use of hot bread is the cause of much indigestion and ill health.

Meats.—Broadly speaking, there are two methods of treating meats. By the first, it is the aim to keep the juices within the meat, as in baking, broiling, and frying. By the second, the object is to extract the juices and dissolve the fiber, as in the making of soups and stews. In order to imprison the juices and thus develop the flavor, the meat must be subjected to intense heat for a short time, so as to coagulate the outer layers of albumen, and afterward a more moderate heat should be employed to complete the cooking. To extract the juices, meat should be cut into small pieces, put into cold water, and slowly raised to the boiling point.

Roasting is probably the best method of cooking meats, especially large, thick pieces. Frying is the worst method, as the heated fat penetrates the meat, dries and hardens it, and renders it indigestible. The American frying-pan is, beyond question, the most deadly instrument that can be named. The sword may claim its thousands, or even its tens of thousands, but the frying-pan numbers its victims by the millions. And yet the skilled French cook robs even this destructive implement of its terror, and furnishes the table not only with meats but with whatever else has been fried, free from soaking grease, finely flavored, and above all, thoroughly digestible. The fault must therefore be ascribed to the cook, and not to the frying-pan.

In an address on "Home Economies Among the Poor People of New York," the Rev. Dr. William S. Rainsford declares that living expenses are entirely too high. "The poor families of New York are in a tight place. Food is not so cheap as it should be. Fish, for instance, should be sold in New York for half its present price.

"Because of these things it is growing more and more difficult for young persons to marry. You have no idea how dangerous this is.

"Another reason for suffering among the poor is that the girls don't know how to cook. One of the best ways to hold even a fairly good man—not a blackguard, but an average man—is to know how to cook.

"This whole country is cursed by bad cooking. It is worse in the rural districts. It makes my heart sick to see the beautiful children, up to ten years, of the Tennessee and Carolina regions, with the shade of frying-pans spreading over their faces, killed by grease—vicious and expensive grease."

In commenting upon the above, a prominent daily says: "Dr. Rainsford is by no means the first man to hold that bad cooking is responsible for many of the sins that men commit. It is well known that a disordered stomach has a corresponding effect upon the brain, causing men to hold views and commit deeds which they would think of only with horror under normal conditions; but this class of missionary work, as it really is, has been much neglected by reformers in the past. They are giving it more attention now, and the cooking-schools, despite the ridicule heaped upon them by the comic writers, are doing good work toward raising the standard of American cooking."

Veal and Pork.—These are regarded as less wholesome than beef or mutton. Both should be well cooked, and ham, sausages, and other forms of pork should never be eaten raw or imperfectly cooked, on account of the danger of introducing the animal parasite which produces in the human body a serious and painful disease known as trichiniasis.

Superfine Flour.—Chemists tell us that the process of bolting removes from the flour not only the outer woody fiber, but also the lime needed for the bones; the silica for hair, nails and teeth; the iron for the blood; and most of the nitrogen and phosphorus required for muscles, brain and nerves; and leaves only the starch which supplies fat and fuel.

Experiments made upon animals show that fine flour alone, which is chiefly carbon, will not sustain life for more than a month, while unbolted flour supplies all that is needed for every part of the body. Wholesomeness and nutrition are sacrificed to that which pleases the eye, alike by the baker and the housewife, so that the fragrant, appetizing bread of our grandmothers is almost unknown.

Potatoes.—Potatoes are largely composed of starch, which supplies only fuel for the capillaries. Analysis shows that they contain only one part in one hundred of muscle-making material, and less than that of phosphorus for brain and nerves.

Animal Food.—Many vegetarians denounce the use of all animal food as constituting an unnatural diet, oppose the slaughter of animals on moral grounds, and declare that vegetables, fruits, and nuts furnish all the elements necessary to the growth, strength, and health of the body.

That a person may subsist, and even be strong and healthy, without the use of animal food is proven by the lives of many vegetarians in all ranks of society. It is recorded of Louis Cornaro, a Venetian nobleman, that for fifty-eight years his daily allowance was twelve ounces of vegetable food and a pint of light wine. In many countries the low wages paid for labor and the high price of meat compel the working classes to depend largely upon a vegetable diet. The Spanish peasant is happy on coarse bread, onions, olives, and grapes. The Italian fares sumptuously on macaroni, polenta, olives, and fruits. Over two millions of people in France and other parts of Southern Europe subsist chiefly on bread made from chestnuts, the annual crop being estimated at fifteen million dollars.

In England and other countries in Northern Europe, the eating of meat is largely a question of wages. With the increase of prosperity, it has been observed, there is a corresponding increase in the use of animal food. In Spain, France, Italy, and the warmer portions of Europe, the cooling acids of the fruits and the less-heating elements of the vegetable kingdom are better suited to the climatic needs of the people.

Probably in no other country is so much meat eaten as in America. The supply here is greater, and wages, as a rule, are better. Many physicians and others interested in domestic science are of the opinion that the health of the people generally, and of those leading inactive or sedentary lives in particular, would be better if less animal food were eaten.

Salted meats are not as nutritious as fresh. The brine absorbs the rich juices of the meat and hardens its fibers. Long-continued use of salt meats, without fresh vegetables, produces scurvy, formerly very prevalent on shipboard, in prisons, and in the army.

Nutrition.—The conversion of food into flesh, bone, brain, and nerve matter, and the other parts of the human body, is comprised in four somewhat distinct processes: Digestion, Absorption, Circulation, and Assimilation. We are apt to think of digestion as a process belonging only to the stomach, but it begins when food is put into the mouth, and continues until the waste is finally excreted from the bowels. The alimentary canal, or food passage, including the mouth, gullet, stomach, small and large intestines, is a tortuous passage, some thirty feet in length.

Mastication.—The first step is that of mastication, or chewing. There are sixteen teeth in each jaw. The front teeth are designed for cutting, and the rough, broad surfaces of the back teeth adapt them for grinding. The structure of the teeth would indicate that man was intended to eat both animal and vegetable food.

The Teeth.—The proper mastication of the food demands that the teeth be kept in good order. After eating, they should be brushed with a soft brush and tepid water in order to remove the particles of food that may be wedged between them or lodged in the crevices. By reason of the heat and moisture of the mouth, these particles soon putrefy, which not only renders the breath unpleasant, but promotes the decay of the teeth.

The enamel, or outer covering of the teeth, if destroyed, is not formed anew. Sharp acids corrode it. Gritty tooth powders, metal tooth picks, and other hard substances scratch or crack it. Sudden changes from hot to cold, in food or drink, tend to destroy it. Do not attempt to crack nuts or hard grains with the teeth.

The Saliva.—The food should not be swallowed until it is thoroughly ground with the teeth. While mastication is in progress, the salivary glands moisten the food and fit it for admission to the stomach. This saliva is the first chemical solvent, and is an important factor in the process of digestion. If the food is not retained in the mouth long enough to become thoroughly ground and properly mingled with the saliva, the work of the stomach will be increased. Persons who bolt their food, and wash it down with water or other liquid, thereby dilute the natural juices of the mouth and stomach, impose upon the latter organ a task for which it is not adapted, and throw the entire digestive machinery out of gear.

The sense of taste being largely dependent upon the saliva, the natural flavors of the food are not fully developed, the food seems insipid, and there is created a taste for pungent sauces and spices which over-excites the digestive organs. Poisonous substances are often swallowed in mistake, which, if retained in the mouth long enough to determine their taste, would be rejected without injury.

The Stomach.—The most important organ of digestion is the stomach. This is a pear-shaped pouch, having a capacity of about three pints. The walls are thin and yielding, and often become unnaturally distended by those who habitually gormandize. Its construction clearly shows that the work of grinding and mashing the food was intended to be performed before it entered the stomach.

The gastric juice, another chemical solvent, is here poured upon the food, which, as rapidly as it is prepared, is passed into the intestines. The time required for the stomach to perform its work varies from one to five hours, according to the quantity and character of the food and the digestive power of the individual. The delicate network of blood vessels which underlies the mucous membrane of the stomach takes up all those elements of the food that are ready to be absorbed.

The Intestines.—The small intestines are continuous with the stomach, and, though very different in shape, are like it in general structure. The bile, which is secreted by the liver, unites with the pancreatic juice, and enters the intestines through a duct about three inches below the stomach. By the joint action of these two fluids, the fatty elements of the food are prepared for absorption. From the mucous membrane, or inner lining of the small intestines, still another juice or fluid flows, whose office is to supplement the work, first, of the saliva in converting starch into sugar; next, of the gastric juice in digesting the albuminoids; and, lastly, of the pancreatic juice and bile in emulsifying the fats. The work of digestion is completed in the small intestines. The indigestible parts of the food are passed into the large intestines, and expelled from the body.

Absorption.—The liquefied food, in its passage through the stomach and small intestines, has been prepared by the various juices for its absorption by the blood vessels and the lacteals, whose minute mouths throng this part of the alimentary canal. The food elements thus absorbed are conveyed to the right auricle, or first chamber of the heart.

Conditions Affecting Digestion.—The quality, quantity, and temperature of the food, and the condition of mind and body, all have an influence upon digestion. In the selection of food, only such articles should be allowed as are fresh, pure, and wholesome. Bread should not be eaten warm. It is more easily digested after being baked a day or two. Flesh of animals recently slaughtered should be thoroughly cooled, and never cooked while yet warm and quivering with life.

Cooking renders many articles of food not only more wholesome and palatable, but also more digestible by reason of the increased temperature. The natural heat of the stomach is about ninety-nine and one-half degrees, at which temperature the operations of digestion are best promoted. Hot soups are therefore a good introduction to the meal. A small glass of ice-water will retard digestion for half an hour.

Sudden joy, anger, grief, or other strong emotion or excitement checks digestion. If the tongue is parched and the mouth dry, the flow of saliva is restrained and the first step in the process of digestion is hindered. The coating of the tongue reflects the condition of the stomach, hence the frequent request of the physician to see the tongue of the patient.

Bodily fatigue destroys appetite and hinders digestion. The expression "I am too tired to eat" is not uncommon.

Intervals for Meals.—Frequent eating is as bad as rapid eating or over-eating. The organs of digestion require periods of rest, in order to renew their strength and restore the juices essential to their perfect operation. No person, except infants and the sick, should require food oftener than once in four hours. If the stomach is in good working order, it will usually complete its task in two hours, unless the food is too great in quantity or too indigestible.

No one should take more than three meals a day, and, to insure sound refreshing sleep and allow the stomach to recover its tone, the last meal should be the lightest and easiest to digest. Dyspeptics and others affected with stomach troubles will find benefit in restricting themselves to two moderate meals a day. Numerous cases are cited of notable cures effected by adopting a regimen of only one meal each day.

Regularity.—Whatever the interval between meals, be it four, five, or six hours, there should be regularity. The stomach, like the mind, forms habits, and the habit of regularity in eating will beget the habit of regularity in digesting and recuperating. The practice of parents in giving children cakes, fruits, and sweetmeats between meals is reprehensible. As a result of habit, many persons grow to feel that a dinner is not complete without a substantial dessert. The mistake consists, not always in the dessert, for that may be as wholesome and nourishing as any part of the meal, but in first fully satisfying the demands of hunger, and afterwards imposing upon the stomach the extra burden of digesting the dessert.

Rest.—For every disease of every organ the first condition is rest. Broken bones and lacerated muscles must have release from active duty or there can be no cure. The vital organs, when diseased, must have all the repose consistent with the operations of life. For affections of the heart, the circulation should be reduced, and all excitement and stimulation to over-action be removed.

Excessive physical or mental exertion, whether immediately before or after meals, interferes with digestion. If before, the energies of the blood will be directed to the part of the body in most active exercise, and cannot suddenly be withdrawn. If after, they will be diverted before having performed their legitimate part in the process of digestion. A short period of relaxation before, and of absolute repose after meals, is most favorable to the proper action of the stomach. The repose should not be carried to the extent of sleeping, for in sleep the stomach, as well as the rest of the body, seeks release from duty.

Drink.—Thirst warns us that the blood is too thick, or that it contains some acrid matter which should be eliminated. Free perspiration makes large demands upon the fluids of the body, and copious draughts of water are required to supply the lack. In this way the system is flushed, the clogged pipes and pores are opened, the waste matter removed, and the system made healthy. In cities the water is usually introduced into houses through lead pipes. Herein lies a danger, and the purer the water and the newer the pipe, the greater the danger. The water gradually corrodes the metal and holds a small quantity of it in solution. After a few months of service, an insoluble coating forms upon the inner surface of the pipe, and protects it from further corrosion. It is a wise precaution to run off the water that has lain in the pipes over night, or during the temporary absence of the family, before using.

Coffee and Tea.—The Americans drink more coffee and the English more tea, *per capita,* than any other nation. As to the wholesomeness of these beverages opinions are greatly at variance. Used in moderate quantities, and especially by persons who lead an active out-door life, no harm is likely to ensue. Many persons drink them for the taste, which is often heightened by the use of cream and sugar, and never stop to question whether they are injurious or otherwise. Such persons usually drink too much. If either produces wakefulness, it should not be used before retiring at night, and if the nerves are unduly stimulated, at any time, its use should be discontinued. Tea should be steeped, not boiled. It contains a certain proportion of tannic acid which is dissolved by boiling, and when drunk, produces a deleterious effect upon the mucous membrane of the stomach, causing dyspepsia with its attendant evils. Children should not be permitted to drink either tea or coffee.

Intoxicants.—While alcoholic preparations may, in rare cases, be prescribed by the physician, their use as a beverage finds no support in science or in experience. There are many who use liquors and tobacco and who yet live to an old age. It is also true that many reach old age without their use. Comparing the lives of a thousand persons who drink and smoke, with a thousand others under the same conditions who do not use liquors or tobacco, it will be found that the latter are not only longer-lived, but are also more healthy. Probably no better test of the question of health and longevity can be found than the experience of the life insurance companies. By them, all intoxicants and tobacco are looked upon with disfavor.

Circulation.—The blood is the most important and the most abundant fluid of the body. It constitutes about one-twelfth of the entire weight of the person. To the eye it appears as a simple fluid, varying in color from a bright scarlet to a dark purple. Under the microscope, it is seen to consist of a clear, colorless fluid in which float a multitude of corpuscles, or solid discs. These corpuscles are so minute that thirty-five hundred, arranged side by side, will extend only one inch, and fourteen thousand, placed one upon the other, would not exceed one inch in height. There are also white corpuscles which are fewer in number, larger, and globular in form.

The size and shape of the blood corpuscles in man differ from those in animals. So important and well-defined is this difference in point of law that the guilt or innocence of criminals has often hung upon the results of a scientific examination of the blood found upon the garments of the suspected person.

Coagulation.—The coagulation, or thickening of the blood, when it leaves the living tissues, is a principle of the greatest importance to life. Without it, the slightest injury might prove fatal. In minor injuries, the blood coagulates, thus closing the mouths of the injured blood vessels, and bleeding ceases spontaneously.

The Heart.—The great center of the circulatory system is the heart. With ceaseless energy it drives the blood through the arteries to every part of the body, laden with the life-giving elements absorbed from the food and vitalized by the oxygen in the lungs. In the outward flow of the blood each part of the body appropriates the particular elements which it requires. The return of the blood through the veins brings with it the waste and cast-off particles of the bones, muscles, and tissues, to be expelled through the lungs, except such elements as exude through the pores of the skin. By this unceasing round of waste and repair, the entire body, it is believed, is renewed every seven years, and some parts are replaced several times within that period. From the moment a human being begins to live, he begins to die.

Action of the Heart.—The alternate contraction and dilation of the muscles of the heart constitute the heart-beats or throbs of the pulse. These vary with the individual. In the average adult, the number of beats is seventy-two per minute. In the cases of Bonaparte and Wellington the number was less than fifty. Heat, food, and exercise increase its action, as cold, fasting, and sleep diminish it. Emotion of joy, grief, and fear also exert a modifying influence.

It is a matter of wonder how the silent forces within a tree can lift from the soil, through its minute pipes, and extract from the air, through the small pores of the leaves, the many tons of material that go to make up the giant of the forest. The tons of physical energy bound up in that small organ, the human heart, is a matter no less marvelous. Estimating the amount of blood expelled by each contraction of the ventricles of the heart at four ounces, we have a total of twelve tons a day, or over four thousand tons in a year.

Assimilation.—The crowning act in the conversion of lifeless food into living tissue takes place in the meshes of the capillary network, and is called assimilation. This process is alike mysterious and wonderful. By a peculiar power of selection, each bone and muscle and tissue appropriates that portion of the blood which it needs for its own development or for the repair of the waste, and applies it in such a manner as to preserve the form and size and strength of the part, ever maintaining a proper balance of the two sides of the body, unless thwarted in its operation by some act of the individual.

Adulteration of Food Products.—National, State, and Municipal Boards of Health, and food inspectors may do much to preserve health, but when they have done all that it is possible for them to do, much will still remain for the individual. With the products of the world exposed for sale in our markets, with the advertising pages of our magazines and newspapers filled with irresistible arguments in favor of some newly-discovered breakfast food or new preparation of canned goods, the need of individual knowledge and caution daily increases.

There is cause for congratulation in the fact that those articles which constitute the larger portion of our food are but little adulterated. In the States that impose legal penalties the proportion of adulterated products is quite low. The value of a stringent law is seen in the decrease of the adulteration of cream of tartar, which, in Massachusetts, fell from forty-two per cent in samples examined in 1879, to five per cent in 1898. Spices, flavoring extracts, and canned goods afford the most promising field for adulteration.

The substitution of ingredients is prompted wholly by a desire for gain, and consists in the substitution of a cheaper for a more expensive article. It is, therefore, a question of ethics rather than of health. If the horse-radish is largely turnip, and the apple-butter chiefly pumpkin, if the currant or raspberry jelly is made of the rich juices of the parings and cores of apples, strained, colored and delicately flavored, who will say that the cheaper fraud is not as wholesome as the more expensive genuine article? In some instances there is an actual advantage to health in the substitution, but this does not justify the deception. Pure, fresh oleomargarine, however wholesome, should not be sold for butter, any more than shoddy cloth should be sold for pure wool.

Dangers to Health.—The contents of tin cans are sometimes affected by the action of the acids upon the tin or the solder. Food should not be allowed to stand in a tin can after being opened. Milk, cream, and butter are quick to take up germs of disease. Scarlet fever and typhoid fever have, in many instances, been traced to this source. The utmost cleanliness and care should be exercised in their handling.

The Diet Cure.—Over-indulgence in eating is the source of many disorders of the system. It is well, at all times, to keep within the limit of the powers of digestion. The way to give the stomach rest is to eat less food and at longer intervals.

Obesity is the result of the accumulation of the fatty properties of the blood in excess of what is needed to repair the waste of the system. The fattening process will be stopped by cutting off the supplies. A restricted diet, the avoidance of fat-producing foods, vigorous perspiration as the result of exercise, and frequent bathing, followed by friction, will be attended by a decided reduction of the superfluous fat. A merchant in England who had reached the enormous weight of four hundred and fifty-seven pounds put himself upon a diet of four ounces of animal food, six ounces of bread, and two pounds of liquid in twenty-four hours. In one week he had reduced his weight thirty pounds, and in six months he had lost one hundred and thirty-four pounds.

In France, there is a method of treatment known as "The Grape Cure." Persons in Paris, broken down by the excitements and dissipations of the city, go off among the vineyards, breathe the pure country air, and live on grapes. From eight to twelve ounces of bread, with grapes at discretion, constitute their daily allowance of food and drink. By this treatment the impurities of the system soon pass off through the kidneys, the bowels, the lungs, and the pores of the skin, and pure, wholesome blood takes the place of that which was diseased.

The Water Cure.—The importance of water can hardly be overrated. No life, whether animal or vegetable, is possible without it. By water all food is dissolved, and so penetrates the system and nourishes the tissues. By water the waste particles of matter are carried off through the skin, the lungs, and the other secreting or excreting organs.

While the waters of many of the spas contain medicinal properties, a large part of the virtue claimed for the springs is due to the free flushing of the system. It is the fad, while sojourning there, to drink frequently and copiously. Any other pure, wholesome water would be nearly, if not quite, as beneficial, if used in the same quantities and under the same conditions.

CLOTHING

Influence of Dress on Health.—While this aspect of the subject of dress receives far less consideration than it deserves, its importance is to be measured only by the importance of human life and by the value that attaches to a state of perfect health. Like fresh air, pure water, and bright sunshine, health is only appreciated when it is gone. The behests of fashion often make sad inroads upon it, but the seductive siren lures us on until we can no longer follow. With scanty strength we then worship at the shrine of Hygeia, but this queenly goddess governs with stern rule, and is often unresponsive to our petitions.

Temperature.—There is a constant interchange between bodies or substances of different temperatures when they are in touch one with the other. The warmer give off heat which is absorbed by the colder, and in this way they tend toward equalization. The normal heat of the average human body is 98.4 degrees, Fahrenheit. When it is exposed to a temperature lower than this, it must be protected by clothing to retard radiation of the body-heat, and thus prevent not only the chilling of the surface but also more serious disorders of the internal organs. In very hot countries, clothing is worn as a protection against heat. The head, especially, needs protection from the sun's rays.

Warmth.—From the standpoint of health, no other property of dress is so important as that of warmth. While certain garments are described as being warm and others as being cool, it is a well-known fact that articles of clothing possess neither warmth nor coolness in themselves. By reason of certain chemical processes constantly going on within the body, there is produced a degree of natural heat, commonly called animal heat.

The body in health seldom varies more than one or two degrees from the normal standard. Conditions of climate, season, exercise, age, or sex have but slight influence upon the average temperature of the body. By conduction, radiation, and evaporation, any excess of heat is quickly reduced. More than seventy per cent of the whole amount of animal heat lost passes through the skin.

Evaporation from the skin is very rapid, and may lead to too sudden cooling of the body. A person who, after exercise that has produced free perspiration, stands in a current of cool air, is apt to take cold. The dryer the atmosphere, the more rapid is the cooling process. The most uncomfortable and oppressive atmospheric condition is that in which the air is heavily laden with moisture and the temperature high. Evaporation from the body is then slow, and the sensation of heat is oppressive.

It is a mistaken notion that clothing keeps the cold out. Its purpose is to keep the heat in, or, in other words, to prevent the rapid radiation of heat. We speak of warm clothing and of cool clothing. That clothing is warm which retards the giving off of heat from the body. The Indian wraps a blanket about his body to keep it warm; we wrap a blanket around a piece of ice to keep it from melting.

Any clothing that prevents the rapid escape of heat from the body is said to be a bad conductor, and is called warm. Woolen textures rank first among dress materials as poor conductors, and are therefore best adapted for winter clothing. Silk and cotton come next. Linen is a good conductor of heat; that is, it carries off the heat from the surface of the body very rapidly, and produces a sensation of coolness; therefore, all dress materials made from flax are said to be cool.

Materials.—The principal materials used for clothing are wool, cotton, linen, and silk. These differ greatly in weight, texture, warmth, porosity, power to absorb moisture, and in other less important qualities.

In a climate so changeable as that which prevails in most parts of the United States, the body, and especially the trunk, should be protected at all seasons from sudden chill by the use of under garments containing wool. Even in the warmest weather it will be found that a light woolen fabric absorbs the perspiration, and is more agreeable to the skin than cotton. The wearing of a flannel band, eight to ten inches in width, buttoned around the waist next to the skin, will prove an excellent protection to the kidneys and the abdominal region. Silk is light and soft, and as it retards the giving out of heat from the body, is worn for under garments, especially by those to whom wool is irritating or otherwise unpleasant. Rubber cloth is useful for rain coats, but as it prevents evaporation of the perspiration, it increases the liability to chill, and renders the wearer uncomfortable except in cold weather.

Animal Heat.—The bird is warmer than the air in which it moves; the fish possesses a higher temperature than the water. As before remarked, chemical changes are constantly going on in the system which give rise to this result. Even plant life is subject to this law. A delicate thermometer placed among a cluster of geraniums about to burst into flower will show a temperature a degree or two higher than the surrounding air.

Warm-Blooded Animals.—Those animals possessing well-developed lungs and large breathing capacity are usually active in movement, and are classed among the warm-blooded animals. They comprise birds, quadrupeds, and man. The animals possessing small lung development are for the most part inactive, and are cold to the touch, indicating a low temperature. Such are the frog, toad, lizard, snake, and tortoise.

These facts show the connection between respiration and animal heat, the temperature being in proportion to the amount of oxygen consumed. Birds have the largest lung development in proportion to size, are most active in movement, and indicate the largest amount of animal heat.

Adaptation to Climatic Conditions.—The Polar bear suffers from the heat of the Temperate zone, and would not survive a week in the Torrid. The African lion would fare no better were he suddenly transported to the Frigid zone. Man alone, of all the animal creation, is able to adapt himself to the extremes of heat and cold. By changing his clothing, shelter, and food, he is able to create for himself an artificial climate wherever he may choose to reside. No Arctic winter has been found too cold for a Peary, Nansen, or Greely to withstand, and no African plain or jungle too hot for a Livingstone or Stanley to explore.

Evaporation.—The temperature of the body is regulated by means of perspiration. Heat induces perspiration, and its evaporation lowers the temperature of the body. Cold retards perspiration, and the heat is retained within. The principle of evaporation is illustrated in the manufacture of artificial ice. Men who labor in glass works, iron and steel foundries, and in the engine rooms of large steam vessels are exposed to great heat, yet enjoy as good health as those who are engaged in other occupations. Persons have been known to remain several minutes in an atmosphere heated above the boiling point, without materially increasing the temperature of their own bodies.

Perspiration goes on continually, night and day. This fact emphasizes the importance of a complete change of clothing upon retiring at night, so that the clothing worn during the day may be thoroughly aired. In like manner, the clothing worn at night, together with the sheets, blankets, and pillows, should be aired, and, if possible, exposed to the sun for a time, before the bed is made up.

Color of Clothing.—The color of our dress is not wholly a matter of pleasure to the eye. In general, it is known that white is cool and black is warm. Scientific experiment has shown that cloth of the same material, when exposed to the rays of the sun, absorbs heat in the following proportions: white, 100 heat units; light yellow, 102; dark yellow, 140; light green, 155; Turkey red, 165; dark green, 168; light blue, 198; dark blue, 206; black, 208. When not exposed to the sun, the color has little or no influence upon the absorption of heat.

The color of underclothing has practically but little influence upon the amount of heat radiated from the body, but the color of the outer dress has much to do with regard to the amount of heat absorbed from the sun's rays.

Absorption of Moisture.—The property of absorbing moisture is of much importance in the hygiene of clothing. The best material for clothing to be worn next to the skin is that which, while retaining the natural heat, or giving it off very slowly, absorbs the moisture from the body, and diffuses it through its meshes. The skin is thus relieved of the cooling effect of this evaporation, which might prove harmful.

Porosity.—The ventilating property of clothing, or the ease with which air passes through its meshes, is called porosity. The most porous of dress fabrics is flannel, which is, at the same time, the warmest. Its porosity, as compared with that of linen, is as 100 to 58.

Impermeability to Water.—As a protection against rain, the simple mackintosh, or the mackintosh cloth, is the best. The latter is more pleasing to the eye, but the outer wool covering absorbs enough moisture to add somewhat to the weight of the garment, which is a slight disadvantage.

All waterproofs present this serious evil, that while they exclude the outer moisture, they prevent the escape of the natural moisture from the surface of the body. This, however, is, generally speaking, a lesser evil than to expose the body to storm and cold, with the risk of serious illness. It is not unusual to add to the waterproof the further protection of an umbrella. In such case, the discomfort of excessive perspiration may be relieved by occasionally loosening a button or two about the neck and chest.

Underclothing.—Taking all things into consideration, wool is, without doubt, the best material for garments worn next to the skin. In cold weather it maintains the natural heat of the body. In warm weather it quickly absorbs the free perspiration, giving off the moisture through its meshes, and thus preventing the too rapid evaporation from the surface of the body, which tends to produce chill and other resulting disorders. It also serves to protect the body from the hot rays of the sun, and from the heat of boilers and furnaces. No other substance so effectually modifies the evil effects of sudden and rapid changes of temperature. In the extreme cold of the polar regions and in the oppressive heat of the tropics, it is alike satisfactory. The thickness of the texture and the closeness of the weave must be determined by the climate and the season.

Disadvantages of Woolen Undergarments.—With all their advantages, woolen undergarments are not wholly free from disadvantages. The most common criticisms are that they are heavy, less cleanly than linen, and they sometimes produce irritation. For an equal weight, wool is the warmest of all dress materials. For summer wear, only that which is thin, light, and loose in web is usually chosen. Light flannel suits have become very fashionable for summer outing, both for men and women.

Woolen undergarments rapidly absorb the excretions from the skin. The water soon evaporates, but the more solid portions are held in the fibers of the garment. Woolen underwear should be washed as frequently as that of cotton, linen, or silk. Unfortunately for the health of the individual, it does not show dirt so quickly as the other materials, and, by the lower classes, is often washed less frequently than it should be.

The therapeutic value of flannel depends in no small degree upon its power to stimulate the skin. It is this that makes it popular with the old, and with those whose circulation is sluggish. For the delicate, the scrofulous, and the rheumatic, flannel undergarments are especially desirable.

Another objection might be urged to the use of woolen underwear, in that it so often shrinks and becomes hard when washed. It is possible, however, to have flannels and other woolen goods come from the wash as soft and light as when they went in. Care should be taken not to subject them to sudden and extreme changes of temperature while washing and drying.

Effects of Tight-Fitting Underwear.—A woolen shirt or undervest, quite loose, will be much warmer than a like garment of the same material, close-fitting. In the loose garment, there is a constant stratum of air between the body and the clothing. This air has almost the same effect as an additional garment. It acts as a non-conducting medium between the surface of the body and the external atmosphere.

Material loosely woven is warmer than the same material closely woven. Clothing worn in successive layers is warmer than the same quantity of material woven in a single layer. Two shirts worn, the one over the other, will afford more warmth than the same quantity of wool or cotton or silk woven into one garment.

Underwear should be light and porous, and permeable to air. Very fine materials densely woven are not so healthful as those that are more open.

Night Attire.—Night is the time for rest, not only from mental toil and physical labor, but also rest for the functions of the body, so far as possible. To this end, it has been recommended that the evening meal be eaten long enough before retiring to enable the digestive apparatus to have completed its work.

For many persons, cotton and linen are found to be more restful, for night wear, than garments made of wool. Even when woolen underclothing is worn with comfort and satisfaction during the day, there is, to some persons, a pricking sensation, a slight surface irritation, in the use of woolen night wear which is destructive of rest. The activities of the skin, as well as the other bodily functions, require a measure of repose.

The old, the delicate, and the very young may use a light woolen night-dress outside that of linen or cotton. If comfort demands the use of wool next to the skin, it should be light in weight, finely woven, and with a smooth surface.

Cleanliness and health alike demand that no part of the clothing worn during the day should be worn while sleeping. The garments worn in the day should be thoroughly aired and dried during the night, and the moisture absorbed by the night clothing should be allowed to evaporate, and the garments ventilated during the day. In cold climates and in cases of sickness, weakness, or of delicate constitution, the dress of the night as well as of the day must be adapted to the requirements of the case.

Hats.—In the advancement from barbarism to civilization, the head was the last part of the body to be covered. Nature originally furnished, in the form of a thick mat of hair, all the covering that was necessary for the head. Baldness was then unknown. While the demands of modern society must be complied with, and hats must be worn, the nearer we can approach to Nature's plan the better.

A hat should be light, loose, and well ventilated. A heavy hat presses with undue weight upon the scalp. A tight-fitting hat interferes with the free circulation of the blood. A hat that is close in its texture, prevents the escape of the heated air within, and not only produces a sense of oppression but is believed to be the most fertile cause of baldness. Silk hats for men are especially objectionable on this ground. All close hats should be supplied with efficient means of ventilation. The head, like any other part of the body, perspires, and if the hat is removed in a cooler atmosphere or in a current of wind, a cold in the head is apt to follow.

The chief cause of baldness is pressure of the hat, which constricts the blood vessels and so interferes with the nutrition of the hair bulbs. It is probable, also, that the shutting off of air and light by the hat promotes baldness. An unhealthy condition of the scalp results, the sign of which is an excess of dandruff.

Baldness is almost unknown among savages, who wear no hats, and is comparatively rare with men in the tropics where very light hats are worn. Laborers are less prone to baldness than business or professional men. They generally wear soft hats or caps, which are often pushed to the back of the head, so that the scalp gets plenty of light and air. There is no good reason why, if properly treated, the hair should not last as long as the man. Wear a soft, loose, well-ventilated hat, and wear it as little as possible, and never keep it on in the office or house.

In hot weather and in tropical climates hats should be of a light color, with a considerable crown and ample brim. In the United States, the ordinary straw hats, if not too closely made, answer every requirement. For the intense heat of Africa or India, more elaborate head-gear is found necessary. The ill effects of special exposure to the sun's heat may be reduced by wearing, in the crown of the hat, a thin sponge, or even a handful of grass or leaves, or other light, porous substance.

From the standpoint of health, but little criticism can be made against the head-gear of women. Nature has provided them with a splendid covering of hair for warmth and protection. The woman's hat, or bonnet, is largely an object of adornment. Fashion, at times, dictates an unequal distribution of its weight, or an over-burden of ornament, or a lack of protection to the eyes, but, for the most part, it is light, loose, and admits of free ventilation. Veils are more or less injurious to the eyes, and if worn so as to cover the nose and mouth, prevent the free escape of the exhalations from the lungs. The dyes used in veils have, in some instances, been productive of face eruptions and other disorders.

The Neck.—The improper clothing of the neck is responsible for much ill-health. The high collars for men, the tight-fitting high collars and neck bands for women, the scarfs, handkerchiefs, and other neck apparel in winter produce an excess of heat. Cold air is inhaled, and the result is some form of sore throat.

Fashion makes greater demands upon the powers of endurance, or resistance, of women than of men. To go warmly clad through the day, and then to put on a ball or party dress, exposing the neck and shoulders to repeated currents of cold air, requires a degree of vitality that many do not possess, and the physician's and undertaker's labors are increased by the victims of fashion.

The neck should be comfortably clad, and kept at the normal temperature as nearly as possible. It is the sudden change from an over-heated neck and chest to that of the opposite extreme that causes the trouble. The boy who, with scarf tightly wrapped about his neck, fights his mimic battle with snowballs until the perspiration flows from every pore, and then throws aside jacket and scarf while he rests, and the girl who, in furs and tippet, skates until she becomes thoroughly heated, and takes off her wraps while she stops to breathe, have many imitators among the older boys and girls in the world.

As to the proper amount of covering for the neck, much depends upon habit, and not a little upon individual requirement. The important point is to preserve uniformity, and to guard against sudden changes. The sailor with neck freely exposed is fully as exempt from colds as is the soldier whose neck is more warmly clad. If they should suddenly exchange their manner of dress, the result would be disastrous to both.

The important blood-vessels that supply the face, head, and brain, and the jugular veins which return the blood to the heart, all pass through the neck. The clothing about the neck should therefore be loose, so as to allow the freest passage of the food, breath, and blood, and the fullest movement of the head.

Male Attire.—While appearance demands that the outer clothing should be neat-fitting, comfort and health require that it should be sufficiently loose to admit of the freest movements of the body. It should be as light as possible to insure proper protection from the cold. Weight does not always count for warmth. Many persons prefer light flannels as outer garments for warm weather.

The trousers should be supported from the shoulders by suspenders. Belts involve more or less constriction of the abdomen, and are injurious. Men suffer greater disadvantage from their use than women. The practice of wearing a belt during the summer months is especially objectionable.

Female Attire.—Healthful and proper clothing implies, (1), the protection of the body against extremes of heat and cold, and the maintaining of an equable temperature in every part; (2), the absence of all superfluous material and needless weight; and (3), the non-interference with the normal functions of the body.

Mrs. Woolson, a writer on Dress and Health, says: The limbs have not half the amount of covering which is put upon the trunk of the body. Many garments have no sleeves, or sleeves that terminate a few inches below the shoulders. As to the legs, the clothing which should increase in direct ratio to the distance from the body to the feet, diminishes in the same ratio. Thin drawers, thinner stockings, and wind-blown skirts which keep up constant currents of air supply little warmth to the limbs beneath. The feet, half-clad and pinched in tight shoes, are chilled in consequence.

The trunk of the body has as many zones of temperature as the planet it inhabits. Its frigid zone is above, on the shoulders and chest; for, although the dress-body extends from the neck to the waist, most, if not all, of the garments worn beneath it are low-necked. The temperate zone lies between the shoulders and the belt, for that region receives the additional covering of undervest, corset, and chemise. The torrid zone begins with the belt and bands, and extends to the limbs below; for all the upper garments are continued below the belt, and all the lower garments come up as far as the belt, so that the clothing over the whole hip region must be at least double what it is over any other section. But it is more than double; it is quadruple, for the tops of all these lower garments have a superfluous fullness of material which is brought into the binding by gathers and plaits.

It will be observed from the above that the three rules laid down for a perfect dress are all violated. First, the unequal preservation of heat; second, the excessive weight, largely supported by the waist; and, third, the constriction of the waist and pressure upon the abdomen caused by the gathering of so many garments at this point.

The Petticoat.—Petticoats are objectionable in several ways. They seriously impede movement. They involve an unnecessary expenditure of muscular force by hampering the action of the lower limbs. They stir up and accumulate the dirt of the streets, or drag through mud and slush, often occasioning wet ankles and engendering disease. Thick woolen drawers reaching to the feet, or, better still, the one-piece underwear which covers the entire body except the head, hands, and feet, would furnish more warmth and distribute it more equally than the "many petticoat" plan, and save the weight and secure freer movement by enabling the wearer to dispense with one or more of these objectionable garments. This would add greatly to the comfort of the wearer, reduce the weight of the nether garments, prevent in large measure the undue heat of the abdominal region, and would not materially change the appearance of the outer dress.

Tight Lacing.—It is said that Hippocrates earnestly reproached the ladies of his time for too tightly compressing their ribs, and thus interfering with their breathing powers. Fashion and Health must be sworn enemies, for they have not come much nearer together since. We smile at the Chinese lady who cramps her foot until it is neither fit to look upon nor to walk upon. Yet, the tortures she endures are no greater than those voluntarily assumed by many American women at the behest of the same tyrant, Fashion.

The unnatural constriction about the waist and abdomen involves every vital function. It compresses the lower part of the lungs, diminishes their capacity, and thus interrupts the proper oxidizing of the blood. It cramps the heart, and often results in fainting and swooning, to say nothing of the more permanent results of impeded heart action. It forces out of shape and place the liver and stomach, restricts the flow of the bile and other stomachic juices, and seriously interferes with the important function of digestion. It restricts the action of the intestines, producing constipation, with all its attendant evils. It presses upon the blood vessels leading to the bowels and the lower extremities, diminishes the circulation, produces cold feet, and often causes varicose veins. And, worst of all, those delicate organs peculiar to women are so crushed by the unnatural pressure, and so obstructed in their normal action, that the function of motherhood is most seriously impaired, the poor deformed woman becomes the victim of untold suffering, and the wretchedness entailed upon the race is widespread and far reaching.

A Deformity.—The devotee of feminine fashion will doubtless resent the intimation that she is deformed, or is likely to become so. A missing finger or hand, a shortened arm or leg, an inverted foot or curved spine—these are set down as deformities. In short, any wide departure from the normal human structure must be classed as a deformity.

The bony framework of the thoracic cavity in its natural shape is an irregular cone, whose apex is at the neck, and whose widest part, or base, is formed by the spread of the lower ribs. By constantly compressing the waist, the flexible lower ribs yield to the pressure, and after a time become fixed in this unnatural position, and that which was the base of the cone becomes the apex, and the widest part is now near the top. From the standpoint of anatomy, the latter condition can be nothing less than a deformity.

Are Corsets Ever Necessary?—For any unnatural or unhealthy conditions, the physician or specialist alone must prescribe. There is no reason why the bones and muscles of a woman, as well as a man's, should not support the upper part of the body without artificial aid. As remarked in another chapter, the body acquires habits. After wearing corsets or stays for a time, their absence will doubtless suggest a lack of support, for the muscles have become weakened from a lack of use.

The skirts and other garments should be supported from the shoulders, and not from the waist. To this end, an under jacket, close-fitting, but in no sense compressing the body, loose in texture so as to be permeable to the air, with straps over the shoulders, should be worn. To this, by means of buttons, all the lower garments should be attached. No steel or other stiff supports should be tolerated. With this system in general use for a generation, the amount of suffering saved would be incalculable, and the advantage to the race would be beyond compute.

The Feet.—In so far as the health is affected by the dress, next to the evils of tight lacing come the evils of tight shoes. The feet being remote from the heart, the circulation of the blood at this point is not as free as in other parts of the body. This in itself tends to beget cold feet, and at once suggests the advantage of warm stockings and stout shoes in order to keep out the cold and wet, and to induce a freer current of warmth-producing blood.

The small foot is almost as much an object of worship as the small waist. The temptation to cramp it by tight and ill-fitting shoes is great, and is not wholly confined to the weaker sex. Large shoes may be ill-fitting and injurious, as well as small ones, often rubbing the skin and producing blisters and sores.

The shoes should be close-fitting but not tight, thus allowing free circulation of air as well as of blood, and also the freest action of the bones and muscles. Like other parts of the dress, the shoes must be adapted to the season. In cold and wet weather the soles should be thick so as to keep out the dampness. The maxim, "Keep the feet warm and the head cool," is none the less good because it is old.

Rubbers.—Tight-fitting rubbers impede circulation, and, on this score, are objectionable. But the disadvantages of wet or damp feet are far greater. Through the winter and spring months the streets and pavements are rarely free from dampness, and light rubbers or sandals should be worn. Persons who are exceptionally susceptible to colds need to be doubly careful to keep the feet dry and warm.

Stockings.—The stockings, too, should be stout and warm. For most persons, wool is the best material. If the rough surface is uncomfortable to the skin, those of a smoother surface may be tried. A thin silk stocking with a woolen one of moderate thickness outside will make no more bulk than a single heavy woolen stocking, and will be found equally warm.

Some persons when about to undergo extreme exposure to cold wrap the feet with a thickness or two of tissue paper, either under or outside of the stocking. Being impervious to the air, paper is not to be recommended for general use.

The physical annoyances and discomforts growing out of ill-clad feet are such as to demand that great care be given to this part of the dress. Corns, bunions, and in-growing nails are so common that it is a rare thing to find a person who is free from these afflictions.

Heels.—Heels of moderate height are desirable. High heels throw the foot into the front of the shoe, cramp the toes, and destroy the natural action of the foot. The French heel, so coveted by many ladies, is an abomination. It is not only too high, but, being placed under the arch of the foot, defeats Nature's purpose in the construction of the arch. Children under twelve years should not wear heels.

Wide Soles.—The width of the sole should always be greater than the width of the foot. With the foot clad in a close-fitting, stout stocking, stand upon a cardboard or piece of stiff paper, bearing the weight of the body upon this foot. With a pencil held in a vertical position, have some one draw the outline of the foot upon the paper. When purchasing a pair of shoes, apply this outline to the soles, and see to it that they are larger at every point than the outline. This will go far toward securing comfort.

Infants require to be warmly clad. The heat-producing powers of the organism are feeble. Clothing should be of a kind and of sufficient quantity to prevent the undue waste of natural heat. Children are often clad too thinly, and exposed to cold before they are strong enough to bear it. The "hardening" process to which some foolish mothers resort is accountable for no small amount of infant mortality. The other extreme is equally reprehensible. Aim to maintain an equable temperature of the room as well as of the body; avoid sudden changes, and keep the child out of draughts. Clothing of fine soft wool, as a rule, is the best.

Evenly Distributed.—The body of the child usually is too warmly clad, while the arms and neck are often insufficiently covered. The long skirts of infants are objectionable because they keep the legs too warm and hamper them in their movements, so essential to their growth and development.

Weight.—The weight of the clothing of all persons, of whatever age, should be as light as is compatible with comfortable warmth, but it is a matter of double importance to infants and young children.

Constriction.—Many young mothers have done their infant children incalculable injury by tightly pinning about their tender bodies the swathing band and the upper parts of the skirts. The heart and lungs, stomach and liver, as well as the rest of the body, need room for growth. Instances are recorded of infants having died from being deprived of sufficient room to breathe properly. Here again, the opposite extreme must be avoided. Socks that come well up on the legs should be provided. The dress should not be so loose about the neck as to admit cold draughts of air to the chest or spine. As with older persons, the petticoats and nether garments should be suspended from the shoulders as soon as the child is old enough to walk. The increase in the average life of the American is largely due to the better care of the children.

BATHS AND BATHING

Why We Bathe.—The first object of bathing is cleanliness. The importance of this object is so widely recognized as to have passed into a proverb, "Cleanliness is next to godliness." A second object of the bath is to stimulate the functions of the skin. A large amount of waste matter is thrown off through the pores, and unless removed by frequent bathing, soon becomes clogged, and sickness ensues. A third object is the pleasurable exhilaration which attends a plunge into the swimming pool, stream, or surf. The street urchin, with no ungovernable desire for cleanliness, and with little thought of the importance of keeping his cuticle in good working condition, plunges into the nearest stream long before the summer days have tempered the water to such a degree as to beguile his older brother.

The Skin.—In order that the advantages of bathing may be fully understood, it is necessary that we have some knowledge of the nature and structure of the outer covering of the body. This garment is soft, pliable, close-fitting, and quite thin, yet sufficiently strong to resist the ordinary contact with surrounding objects.

The skin is composed of two layers, the outer, called the epidermis, or cuticle, and the inner, called the cutis, or true skin. The two layers are closely united. When, from a burn or other cause, a blister is formed, a watery fluid separates the cuticle from the true skin.

The cuticle is very thin, and is composed of minute flat cells, arranged layer upon layer. These, as they are worn out, fall from the body in the form of fine scales. When the cuticle in the palms of the hands or other parts of the body is subjected to severe pressure, or friction, it becomes thick and hard, and better adapted to manual labor.

The cutis, or true skin, is firm, elastic, and very sensitive. Its surface is covered with minute elevations called *papillæ*. These contain the blood vessels which supply the waste of the skin, and also the nerves which are largely concerned in the sense of touch.

Its uses.—The skin, which seems like a very simple membrane in structure, is, in reality, a very complex and elaborate organ. With its numerous blood-vessels, lymphatic vessels, and nerves; its millions of *papillæ* and pores and sweat ducts; its innumerable hair-follicles with their sebaceous glands and muscles; its odoriferous glands and special pigment-bearing cells, it is well equipped to perform the various duties assigned it.

First, it serves to protect the softer parts of the body which lie underneath it. Secondly, it regulates the temperature of the body by preventing, on the one hand, the too rapid radiation of natural heat, and, on the other hand, by reducing the temperature through the process of perspiration. Thirdly, through its millions of pores, it is constantly throwing off the useless materials found in the excretions of the perspiration and the sebaceous glands.

In order that the skin may perform its functions properly, it must be perfectly clean, the pores must be kept open, and the sweat glands free to throw off all the effete matter and prevent its accumulation within the system. While soap and water are necessary and helpful, free perspiration induced by vigorous bodily exercise or artificial heat will also enable the glands to cast off the more solid substances which accumulate at the bottom.

An eminent French physician has discovered that the annoying odors from the skin which characterize certain persons have their seat in the bottom of the sweat sack, and can be successfully removed by free perspiration followed by a bath.

In addition to the general benefits to the health, of systematic, vigorous exercise and the bath, they will give freshness of color to the skin, prevent the coming of wrinkles, and give to the face a beauty such as no paint or powder can approximate. If ladies with sallow complexions and shrunken countenances would substitute exercise and bathing for facial massage, the benefits of which last only so long as its use is continued, the results would be much more satisfactory.

Many of the common diseases of the skin which destroy the beauty of the complexion are believed to be due to certain microbes. If the skin were kept, by exercise and bathing, in a thoroughly healthy condition, these microbes would find no lodgment, or, gaining a temporary foothold, would readily yield to judicious hygienic treatment.

The Hair and Nails.—These, properly considered, are appendages of the skin. The hair follicles are hollow receptacles, from the bottom of which the hair grows. Alongside each hair follicle are two glands, called the sebaceous glands, which provide the hair with a natural oil or grease, and prevent excessive dryness. This sebaceous matter tends to keep the skin flexible, and serves to protect both skin and hair from the acridity arising from perspiration. The hair serves as a protection, shielding the brain from extremes of heat and cold, and moderating the force of blows upon the head.

The nails not only serve as a protection to the ends of the fingers, but also enable us to grasp more firmly, and to pick up small objects. Well-kept nails contribute much to the beauty of the hand. They are not only an indication of cleanliness but also a mark of refinement.

The Perspiratory Glands.—The skin is provided with numerous sweat-glands which consist of very small tubes with globe-like coils at their deeper extremity. It is estimated that there are 2,800 of these glands to the square inch of the surface of the body.

These glands or pores of the skin are, day and night, constantly excreting a watery fluid. Ordinarily this evaporates as rapidly as it is formed, and the process is called insensible perspiration. Under the influence of heat or exercise the flow is more abundant, and appears upon the surface of the body in the form of minute, colorless drops. This is known as sensible perspiration.

This excretion consists of about ninety-eight parts of water and two parts of solid matter. The quantity of perspiration varies with the temperature, the occupation of the individual, and other circumstances. In an adult, the daily amount is about thirty ounces, or more than nine grains a minute.

Benefit of Perspiration.—Besides freeing the blood of a large amount of water, with the effete matter it contains, perspiration serves to reduce the temperature of the body. This function is most active in hot weather, and the cooling process is proportionally increased, thereby contributing to the comfort of the individual. A partial or temporary check of this excretion is usually attended with headache, fever, and other unpleasant symptoms, and its total interruption is fatal. For the purposes of experiment, rabbits and other small animals have been covered with a coating of varnish, and death invariably ensued in from six to twelve hours.

Importance of Bathing.—As the watery portion of the perspiration evaporates, the solid matter is left on the surface of the skin, and soon clogs the mouths of the pores. The scales of the worn-out cuticle also accumulate, and further impede the action of the skin. These impurities must be removed, not only from motives of cleanliness but also from considerations of health.

General Effects of the Bath.—Bathing, in every form, increases the activity of the internal machinery. It increases the rate of respiration, the activity of the heart, the rapidity of the circulation, the combustion in the tissues, and the perspiration through the skin. This increased activity causes a degree of exhaustion, and makes demand upon the vital forces. The reaction that follows more than restores the depleted vitality, and the bath serves as a tonic to the system.

A Satisfactory Experiment.—A prominent Philadelphia merchant gives the following as a result of his experience: "For a number of years I was troubled with indigestion, and a feeling of general depression. My muscles were soft and flabby, and I was easily fatigued. I was seldom free from colds and their many discomforts. Although there were several gymnasiums near my place of business, I felt that I could not take the time for practice. My condition gradually grew worse, and the drugs and medicines I took did me no good. In sheer desperation, I concluded to see what a little exercise and bathing would do. I chose the early morning and the late evening, as interfering least with business. Upon rising in the morning, and with slight encumbrance of clothing, I devote fifteen minutes to such simple body movements as give exercise to the muscles of the arms, legs, upper and lower trunk, and expand the chest. Then I stand in the bath tub, and with a large sponge filled with cold water, I quickly drench the head, neck, chest, and every part of the body, and, after drying with a soft towel, I give myself a vigorous rubbing with a coarse towel, which produces a delightful glow that lasts for several hours. At night, just before retiring, I again devote ten or fifteen minutes to exercise, and enjoy sound refreshing sleep.

"Since I began this plan of exercise and bathing, some five years ago, my digestion has been excellent, and I enjoy my meals, and seldom ask myself whether it is safe for me to eat this or that, as I used to do. I accomplish much more labor, with less fatigue than formerly, and with none of the old-time languor and depression. My mind is clear and alert, and to my cold sponge bath I ascribe the fact that I rarely have a cold."

Temperature of the Body.—By a wonderful provision of nature, the temperature of the surface of the body is preserved at about 98.4 degrees Fahrenheit, whether the individual resides in the arctic regions or within the limits of the torrid zone. The range of the internal heat of the body is not very great. A deviation of seven degrees from the normal is dangerous. If the temperature of the body rises to 109 degrees or falls to 76, death is almost sure to follow.

Temperature and Kinds of Baths.—From the standpoint of temperature, baths may be classed as hot, warm, tepid, cool, and cold. A hot bath has a temperature ranging from 98 degrees to 112 degrees Fahrenheit; a warm bath from 92 degrees to 98 degrees; a tepid, from 85 degrees to 92 degrees; a cool bath from 60 degrees to 75 degrees; and a cold bath from 60 degrees down to the freezing point of water.

Tepid, warm, and hot baths are employed, not only for cleansing the body, but to diminish blood pressure and to reduce nervous excitability. The hot bath is used in restoring warmth to the body in certain cases of shock, and to remove the effects of exposure to a low temperature.

When the water is of about the same temperature as the body, the effects are neither stimulating nor depressing. In some forms of sleeplessness, a tepid bath taken just before retiring has been found to be effective. In such cases, the body should be covered by the water for ten or fifteen minutes, and quietly dried with a soft towel, without vigorous rubbing or friction.

Hot Bath.—The cold bath stimulates, the hot bath facilitates function. Both hot and cold baths increase the combustion going on within the body. The immediate effect of a cold bath is to chill the surface of the body. This sensation is promptly conveyed by the nerves of the skin, through the spinal cord, to the brain. Respiration and circulation are at once increased, and the temperature of the interior of the body is raised.

The effect of a hot bath is to raise the temperature of the surface of the body and the temperature of the blood. As in the case of a cold bath, the respiration and pulse are quickened, and the escape of carbonic acid from the lungs is increased.

Warm baths can be borne for a longer time than cold baths, but if the temperature be very high they deplete the system rapidly, and faintness is apt to occur. The warm or hot bath leaves the skin in a very delicate condition, susceptible to chill from exposure followed by internal congestion. The bather should dress quickly after a warm or hot bath, and spend a half hour or more in a warm room so as to allow the body to assume its normal temperature, or he may go from the bath to bed, and cover up well.

Popular Error.—The belief is current that it is extremely dangerous to enter a cold bath when the body is heated or perspiring. The bracing effects of the bath are most manifest if taken while the individual is warm. The clothing should be removed quickly, the plunge or douche boldly taken, and immediately followed by a vigorous rubbing with a coarse towel.

Some years ago, an eminent physician, desiring to test the effects of the cold bath when the body is warm, made a series of observations upon himself. The following is his statement: "Every afternoon a free perspiration was produced by a brisk walk in the sun. As soon as the clothing could be cast off, and while the body was still freely perspiring, a plunge was taken into a fresh water bath of about 60 degrees Fahrenheit. No ill result followed. On the contrary, the sensation which immediately followed the bath, and which continued for six or eight hours afterward, was exceedingly pleasant. The health remained perfect, and the weight decidedly increased during the two months the practice was continued. There is probably no danger to a healthy person in this practice, but it is considered advisable to immerse the head first, to avoid increasing the blood pressure in the brain too greatly, which might result if the body were gradually immersed from the feet upward."

The douche consists of a stream of water, hot or cold, which is made to strike the body with force. Its value consists partly in the impact of the water, and partly upon its temperature. It is an exhaustive method of treatment, and must be used with caution.

The Scottish Douche consists in the use of alternating streams of hot and cold water, which produces a powerfully stimulating action. Hot and cold affusion are mild forms of the douche.

The Shower Bath differs from the douche in the division of the streams of water, causing it to strike the body with less force. This method, too, should be used with caution, especially by persons who are not robust.

The Needle Bath is a form of fine shower bath. The bather stands within a coil of pipes perforated with very small holes through which the finely divided streams of water impinge upon every part of the body.

The Vapor Bath combines the two agents, warmth and moisture. The patient sits in a small cabinet or other confined space, into which steam from a boiler or kettle is conducted. In some instances, the head is enclosed so that the vapor may be breathed, but more frequently the head and face are shut out from the vapor-inclosed chamber. The vapor bath can be borne much better than the water bath, the temperature often ranging from 120 degrees to 150 degrees Fahrenheit. Various forms of steam or vapor cabinets are advertised in the popular magazines at small prices. The Russian Vapor Bath consists of a vapor bath of high temperature, followed by a cold douche, and is useful where a quick reaction is desired. The Galvanic Bath and the Electro-magnetic Bath consist merely of a bath of water through which a gentle current from a battery is passed. This is so arranged that the current passes from the water through the body, and affords a powerful stimulant to the skin.

Various forms of medicated baths are employed for specific purposes, but these should not be used except upon the advice of a physician.

Air Bath.—The Hot Air Bath, since the days of ancient Rome, has been not only a popular luxury but also a means of treating disease. Unclad, the bather sits in a room heated to a temperature of 120 degrees to 150 degrees. A glass of cold water is sometimes taken to stimulate free perspiration, after which the bather reclines on a marble slab and is shampooed by an attendant. The body is then thoroughly washed with hot water, and rubbed down with a horse-hair glove. This is followed by a cold shower-bath or douche, after which one is rubbed dry, dresses, and reclines for half an hour on bed or couch.

Sun Bath.—The value of sunshine to animal and vegetable life is apparent to all. Plants become blanched and tender, and lack hardihood, if left without sunlight. Fishes in the subterranean lakes are dwarfed, and have no eyes. Tadpoles kept in the dark never develop into full-grown frogs. Men, growing up in mines or in dark prison cells, are sallow and ill-formed. When Fashion smiles upon brown arms and a tanned face, health is improved, and the darker skin is rendered more hardy and better able to resist exposure.

Sand Baths have, at different times, been held in high esteem. The patient is buried in sand, except his head, and exposed to the full rays of the sun. The surface irritation caused by the sand, combined with the effect of the heat, produces a copious perspiration.

Mud Baths and Pine Baths are popular in parts of Germany. In the former, the body of the patient is imbedded, for a time, in the thick paste or mud deposited by some of the mineral springs, or formed of a mixture of moor-earth and water. In the Pine Baths, a strong decoction is made of the fragrant limbs and tops of the resinous pine trees, which, blended with water, has a stimulating action on the skin.

Surf Bathing.—Sea bathing is more invigorating than fresh water bathing. Persons who cannot bathe in fresh water are often benefited by surf bathing. The stimulating action of the salt water, the impact of the waves, the exhilaration and excitement occasioned by the incoming breakers, and the wholesome exercise which usually attends a sea bath, all contribute to the benefit of surf bathing.

While the danger of chilling and taking cold are less in sea bathing, yet the usual precautions should be observed. If warm, do not wait to cool off before going into the water. This is always hazardous. Plunge boldly in, taking care to wet the head, neck, and face as quickly as possible. Exercise to keep up the circulation. Dive through the rollers, or jump up to prevent being overwhelmed by them. If, after being in the water a few minutes, there is a growing sense of chilliness which cannot be overcome by exercise, the bather, for his own safety, should withdraw at once, however enjoyable the occasion, and seek comfort in dry, warm clothing. A prolonged stay at the sea-shore will enable him to renew his bath daily, and gradually increase its length. At most, it should not exceed thirty minutes. Persons of vigorous constitution may take two dips a day with advantage. A short rest should follow the bath, whenever possible. But if reaction is not established by rubbing and putting on dry clothing, it should be restored by taking a short brisk walk before the rest.

Salt-Water Bath at Home.—Aside from the tonic effects of the sea-air, and the absence of business anxiety and the change in food and habits which a temporary residence at the sea-side involves, a good substitute for the sea-bath may be had by the use of an inexpensive preparation of salt which may be found at almost any drug store.

Reaction.—The phenomenon commonly known as reaction, which accompanies both hot and cold bathing, is quite remarkable. Experiments have shown that if the temperature of a healthy person be raised or lowered by bathing, the subsequent reaction will restore the equilibrium by supplying the loss or withdrawing the excess. Thus nature seems to resent any interference with her normal functions. A German scientist subjected a robust patient to a series of baths of a temperature of 50 degrees Fahrenheit, each lasting twenty-five minutes. The rapid abstraction of heat produced chilliness and shivering, which lasted for several hours after each bath, but this was followed, after an interval, with such an increase of temperature as precisely compensated for the previous loss, and thus the average normal temperature was maintained.

The chronically ill may be divided into two general classes, the one made up of those individuals whose vitality suggests the possession of strong powers of reaction, and for whom the system of heroic treatment, vigorous exercise, cold baths, surf bathing, and sea air are best adapted; the other requiring gentle treatment, much indulgence, mild climate, warm baths, and mountain air.

Frequency of the Bath.—The physical condition of the bather must always be regarded as an important factor in determining the kind of bath, the length of time it should consume, and the frequency with which it should be repeated.

A brisk, cold bath to tone up the system, prevent colds, stimulate digestion, and promote circulation may be taken daily. For many persons, the most convenient time is just after rising in the morning. Fifteen minutes of vigorous exercise before the bath will add to its advantages.

Hot baths, if prolonged, are debilitating and should be taken less frequently. To clean out the pores and remove the excretions and dead cuticle from the surface of the body, two thorough hot baths a week will, for most persons, be sufficient. Some persons get on very well with only one, especially in the winter season when perspiration is less active. The dust, grime, and soil, resulting from one's daily toil, must be removed from hands, face, and body, as often as occasion requires. For this purpose, a basin of warm water and soap will be found sufficient.

Many weakly babes have been sacrificed to their mothers' vanity by subjecting the little ones to the exhausting process of two or three elaborate baths and costly toilets each day. Boys living near ponds, creeks, or rivers often waste their physical forces by spending a large part of the warm summer days in the water. They go in too frequently and remain too long. A morning swim of half an hour, or two dips, one in the forenoon and another in the afternoon, of twenty minutes each, is as much as the strongest boy should take.

Regularity.—In bathing, as in exercise, regularity and system should control, if any physical advantage is expected to follow. A bath now and then, when it happens to suit the convenience of the bather, will not tone up the system nor fortify it against colds. A daily cold bath is best. If that is impossible, it should be taken at least three or four times a week.

Best Time for Bathing.—As remarked elsewhere, every form of bath makes greater or less demand upon the vital forces, and some forms are quite exhausting. It is therefore proper to consider the most suitable times for bathing. It is best not to take a bath when the body is much exhausted, nor to engage in intense physical or mental exercise immediately after a bath.

Under no circumstances should a bath be taken directly after a full meal. Generally speaking the most appropriate time is from two to three and a half hours after a meal, preferably near the noon hour.

For the cold bath, taken quickly, no time is better than just after rising. A warm bath just before retiring will quiet the nerves and assist in producing sleep.

The Value of Soap.—The eminent chemist, Liebig, asserts that the civilization of a nation is high in proportion to the amount of soap it consumes, and that it is low in proportion to its use of perfumes. The cleanliness and refinement of an individual may be measured by the same test. Soap removes impurity; perfume is often employed to conceal it.

Many soaps are positively injurious to the skin. In this, as in other matters, judgment and caution must be exercised. A free use of a good skin soap, with warm or hot water, may be recommended for the weekly or semi-weekly bath when the primary object is cleanliness. The soapy lather should be vigorously rubbed over the body, by the hand or a small coarse towel, so as to remove all excretions from the pores, all greasy deposits of the sebaceous glands, and all dead scales from the cuticle.

This lather must be carefully rinsed off before rubbing with the towels. For the cold tonic and other baths, it is better not to use soap.

Cosmetics.—The use of cosmetics for the complexion is a fertile source of disease. Many of these preparations contain lead and other poisonous mineral substances. The skin readily absorbs these, and the most distressing conditions often ensue.

Hair-dyes also contain lead and other objectionable ingredients. Although less harmful than cosmetics, being generally kept away from the skin, they rob the hair of its lustre and vitality, and should be avoided.

Caution.—Bathing, whether for cleanliness or for recreation, is a most healthful exercise, yet certain precautions are necessary.

1. Avoid bathing within two and a half hours after a meal. The sudden interruption of the process of digestion, especially by a cold bath, is apt to produce nausea. Cases of drowning, usually ascribed to cramps, have been due, in some instances, to interrupted digestion.

2. Avoid bathing when exhausted by fatigue, or from any other cause.

3. Avoid bathing when the body is cooling after perspiration.

4. Avoid bathing in stream or surf if experience proves that after being a short time in the water, there is a sense of chilliness, with numbness of the hands or feet.

5. Avoid chilling the body by sitting or standing undressed, either before going into or coming out of the water.

6. Avoid remaining too long in the water. Rub briskly and dress quickly upon the first sensation of chilliness.

7. The best time for bathing is two or three hours after breakfast. The vigorous and strong may safely take a cold bath before breakfast; the weakly and the young should not attempt it.

8. Those who are subject to dizziness or faintness, should not bathe in stream or surf without first consulting a physician.

9. Avoid a warm or hot bath, if liable to be exposed to a low temperature within two or three hours after the bath.

10. Women should carefully consult their physical condition before venturing to take a cold bath.

11. All persons suffering from organic heart disease should avoid surf bathing.

PHYSICAL EXERCISE

Physical exercise is necessary to the preservation of the health and the cultivation of the strength of the body. By the contraction of a muscle, the circulation of the blood is stimulated, and demand is made upon the supply of food material to replace that which has been consumed. The action of the respiratory process is accelerated, a larger quantity of air is taken into the lungs, more oxygen is absorbed by the blood, and greater tone is imparted to the system. Perspiration is also promoted, effete matters are expelled through the pores of the skin, and the general health is improved.

Definiteness of Purpose.—The person who doesn't know where he is going, never gets there. Know what you are going to do, then do it. There are about four hundred muscles in the human body. It is clearly evident that they cannot all be trained at the same time, nor is it necessary or even desirable that they should be. Those exercises having the most direct bearing upon the specific needs of the individual will naturally come first. If he is troubled with indigestion, two-thirds of the time that he allows himself for daily exercise should be given to remedying that defect, and the rest to supplying some other important need which will bring into play a different set of muscles. If his lung capacity is inadequate, the larger share of time should be given to the correction of this weakness. If shortness of breath and interference with heart action are occasioned by increasing fleshiness, the reduction of his superfluous fat must receive first consideration.

The important thing is to determine what is most needed at any stage of the work, and to strike directly at that point. As, one after another, the special points of weakness are covered, the exercises will gradually take on more and more of an all-round character. As so many of the infirmities of the flesh have their rise in impaired digestion, imperfect respiration, or sluggish circulation, the exercises having relation to these three subjects will always claim attention, not only to secure but also to preserve health.

Mind Engaging.—While those whose mental energies have been on a strain may find relief in exercises somewhat automatic, the most beneficial and satisfactory results, as a rule, are obtained when the mind is kept on the alert and the eye is brought into active play, as in fencing and sparring, or when the exercise contributes to the enjoyment of the individual, and is not self-imposed as an irksome task or an unpleasant duty. The presence and co-operation of a congenial friend adds much to the value of the exercise. Where this is not convenient, the drill should be so varied in kind and in degree, from day to day, as to sustain the interest. Without this, the exercises are apt to be abandoned, or, if continued, they will not be attended with the best results.

Intensity.—Much valuable time is wasted by persons who engage in a certain kind of exercise, not because they are interested in it, but because it happens to be the fad. Whether it be walking, running, swimming, golf, tennis or croquet, they go at it in such a feeble, listless manner as to excite pity rather than enthusiasm.

It is said of President Roosevelt that the only exercise he really enjoys is of that strenuous character which, to most men, would be hard work. Gladstone could give him no points in felling trees, and the cowboys of the plains, after numerous tests, were satisfied that he wore the title of "Rough Rider" by right. It was on one of his western hunting trips that he went two days with two ribs broken, not deigning to mention the circumstance lest it might offend cowboy etiquette to speak of such insignificant matters amid the excitement of the final round-up.

Few men carry the burden of a weightier responsibility than the President, or have more exacting demands made upon their time. No one would have a better right to plead pressure of business as an excuse for taking no physical exercise. On the other hand, no one has greater need of a strong body and a clear brain. Appreciating this fact, his vigorous ride on horseback becomes almost as indispensable as his meals or his sleep, and it is rumored that this is often supplemented by a quiet bout with the gloves. Remembering that, as a child, his body was rather frail, his present rugged health bears strong testimony to the value of persistent vigorous exercise.

Walking.—Rapid walking is one of the best methods of physical exercise. It not only develops the muscles of the legs and thighs, but increases the capacity of the chest. One of its chief advantages is that it is an out-door exercise. Running is still more stimulating, and gives increased activity to the muscles of the limbs and body, and to the organs of respiration.

By combining walking and running with some simple form of in-door exercise, as dumb-bells, Indian-clubs, or pulley weights, a person will have nearly all the advantages of a fully-equipped gymnasium.

Over Exertion.—Severe labor and violent exercise should be avoided. Many cases of broken-down health are due to excessive strain, the result of track races on wheel or foot, and similar indiscretions.

Age, Occupation, and Habit.—Physical exercises must be chosen with reference to the age, occupation, and habit of the individual. The young, the middle-aged, and the old will each, as a rule, require some direction as to kind, and some modification as to length and intensity, of the exercise.

Childhood and Youth.—Healthy children are never at rest except when asleep. This is the prompting of their nature. Their games and plays should therefore be directed, but not too much restrained. If, however, the natural increase in size and weight of a child's body does not keep pace with its years, it would be well for the parent to inquire whether that result is due to excessive exercise, or to some other cause.

Proper habits of sitting, standing, and walking, if not attained during youth, are rarely acquired afterward. The habit of a graceful carriage and a manly or womanly bearing should be established before the age of sixteen. But the exercises that most closely affect the health are those which relate to the expansion of the chest. The lungs vitalize and purify the blood. The larger their capacity, the more satisfactorily will they accomplish their work. With a good supply of pure blood, the growth and health and vigor of the body will be largely provided for.

Middle Life.—While judgment and discretion in the kinds of exercises, and in the manner of doing them, are, at every period of life, desirable, persons from 20 to 35 years of age are able to undertake severer tasks and to withstand greater shocks to the system than the young or the old. Persons from 35 to 50 years of age may take long walks but should be cautious about rapid running. At this age exercises requiring endurance and persistence are better than those demanding intensity or violence. This is especially applicable to those whose occupation is sedentary. Any hereditary tendency to disease is apt to show itself during this period, and should be carefully watched by the individual and by his physician, for by it the kind and degree of the exercise should be determined.

Old Age.—Unless the habit of taking physical exercise has been pursued more or less constantly through life, persons in advanced years, especially if feeble, need to observe great caution in beginning it, on account of the unusual strain upon the heart and blood-vessels. Their native power of resistance being small, any severe shock or strain upon the system may be attended with serious results. William Cullen Bryant, at eighty years of age, took an hour of severe exercise, followed by a cold bath, before breakfast, then walked three miles to his office and back again, in all states of weather, but he had kept up his physical training through life, and found in it a pleasure as well as a benefit to health.

With increasing years, the duties and responsibilities of the busy man increase. Instead of the walk or the ride on horseback, the stately coach, which more fittingly represents his growing wealth, is now used for his afternoon recreation, the coachman relieving him of even the mental and physical stimulus of driving. Wealth is a menace to health, so far as it tends to discourage the simple living upon which health depends.

A much wiser course would be to keep the human machinery oiled and in good condition, by systematic exercise. Hinges of iron and steel must be oiled and used to keep them from creaking and rusting. The membrane that secretes the lubricating fluid and supplies it to the opposing surfaces of the bones and to the ligaments which surround them is stimulated to activity by the motion of the joint itself. Stiffening joints, sluggish circulation, and torpid liver are the sure penalties of inactivity.

Some years ago, two prominent business men, one sixty-four, the other sixty-three years of age, engaged in a walking contest. The younger walked 209 miles, the older 211 miles in three and one-half days, an average of sixty miles a day. James Russell Lowell was unwilling to ride when he could possibly walk. Gladstone was famous as an ax-man as well as a statesman, and continued this exercise nearly to the end of his life. Instances of great mental activity after seventy are almost invariably those of men who have kept up since early manhood a constant habit of vigorous daily exercise. It is only in this way that the arteries are kept from hardening, and that the brain is kept supplied with the blood to renew its cells.

Physical Culture for School Children.—In childhood and youth, bad habits are easily corrected and good ones established. If the chest is weak and flat, this is the time to remove the defect. If one shoulder is a trifle higher than the other, correct the default before it becomes confirmed. Build up the arms and shoulders and chest to be strong and well shaped. It is in youth, while the bones are elastic, that the perfect frame must be built. Accustom the muscles of the trunk and limbs to healthy and graceful action. This becomes easy and natural, when given proper direction, and will result in making a vigorous, well-built man or woman, capable of meeting the difficulties and discharging the duties that come alike to all.

Over-Study.—A prominent magazine recently devoted a page to brief statements of parents, teachers, and physicians, testifying in eloquent but most pathetic terms to the crying evils of over-study and the lack of physical recreation. In reply to the questions asked, one physician says, "Twelve children are under my professional care from over-study."

Another writes, "During the last school year I treated over forty children suffering from over-study. In more than thirty of the cases I had to advise withdrawal from school."

A parent says, "We have four daughters, and had to take all of them out of school."

From the sufferers themselves we have, "At seventeen I broke down. Today, at thirty, I am still an invalid."

"For twelve years I, a young woman, have tried to overcome nervous prostration, directly brought on by over-study."

"Pushed beyond my endurance as a child, I am to-day a nervous mother with children so nervous that it is pitiable."

"An ambitious father caused me to be shattered in nerves before I was sixteen. My bed has ever since been almost my constant companion."

The Remedy.—In the face of the above deplorable facts, it is evident that, with all our boasted improvement in the system of education, there is something sadly lacking. Proper attention given to physical exercise and recreation, with sufficient time for sleep, would have saved the lives and established the health, not only of the few cases above cited, but of thousands of others as well.

Physical Education Compulsory.—Physical culture should be made compulsory in every school in the land. The teacher should be as fully equipped in this as in any other department of his work. In cities and in towns of considerable size the matter should be under the direction of a competent specialist, who would infuse life and energy into the work, and hold the teachers to their duty. Shirking, whether by teachers or scholars, should be strictly prevented. Fifteen minutes, twice a day, in the lower grades, and thirty minutes, once a day, in the upper grades, would serve to put the children in good physical condition.

Caution.—The enthusiasm and alacrity with which children take hold of physical training afford encouragement to the doubting teacher, and, at the same time, prove the need of constant watchfulness. Suppose, in a class of forty, one-fourth of them have flat, weak chests. These should be formed into a special class, and ten minutes a day devoted to the one purpose of enlarging the chest. Begin very mildly, so that the weakest chest will experience neither pain nor ache from the exercise. Repeat this work daily for a week, without increase, and do not miss a stroke. Miss any other drill rather than this. The second week, the exercises may be made a trifle harder, or longer, or both. If apparatus is used, see to it that the pupils do not get hold of heavy pieces, or attempt more difficult exercises than they are prepared for. Overdoing here is as bad as over-study. Strict discipline must be preserved, and the same thoughtful attention given to this as to any other department of study.

Illustrations of the Results of Physical Training.—Wherever physical education has been tested in the schools, of whatever grade, and in whatever country, the results have furnished the most abundant proof of its value. Doctor Sargent, one of the most eminent instructors in physical education in this country, gives the results of six months' training with a class of two hundred young college men, devoting to it only one-half hour a day, four times a week. The only apparatus used was light dumb-bells, Indian-clubs, and pulley-weights. The average age was 18.3 years. The average increase in height was one-fourth of an inch; in weight, two pounds; in chest (contracted), ¾ inch; in chest (inflated), 1¾ inches; in girth of forearm, ¾ of an inch; of upper arm, 1 inch; in width of shoulders, ¾ inch; in girth of hips, 2¼ inches; of thigh, 1½ inches; of calf, ¾ inch.

Prof. Maclaren, of England, gives the results of four and one-half months' training, with a class of boys from the Royal Military Academy, ranging in years from sixteen to nineteen. The increase in height was from 1 to 1¾ inches; in weight, from 1 to 8 pounds; in girth of chest, from ½ to 5¼ inches; forearm, from ⅛ to ½ inch; upper arm, from ½ to 1⅝ inches. With a class of older persons, nineteen to twenty-eight years, he reports the largest gain in weight, 16 pounds, with an average gain of 10 pounds; in girth of chest, 5 inches, with an average of 2⅞ inches; of forearm, 1¼ inches, with an average of ¾ inch; upper arm, 1¾ inches, with an average of 1¹¹/₁₆ inches. These gains were made in 7⅔ months.

Prof. Maclaren gives a humorous account of twelve non-commissioned officers who had been selected from different branches of the service, and sent to him to qualify as instructors in the British Army. These men ranged in years from nineteen to twenty-nine; in height, from five feet five inches to six feet; in weight, from 128 to 174 pounds, and all had seen service. He says, "The muscular additions to the arms and shoulders, and the expansion of the chest were so great as to have absolutely a ludicrous and embarrassing result. Before the fourth month, several of the men could not get into their uniforms without assistance, and when they had got them on, they could not get them to meet by a hand's breath. In a month more, they could not get into them at all, and new clothes had to be procured, pending the arrival of which the men had to go to and from the gymnasium in their great coats. One of these men had gained five inches in actual girth of chest." In the case of the youngest, he reports "a readjustment and expansion of the osseous framework upon which the muscles are distributed."

This case is important as proving that proper physical exercise will materially change even the bony structure of the body. What a source of comfort and encouragement to the young man or woman who is hollow-chested, and who considers himself or herself a marked victim of that dread disease, consumption.

Need of Exercise for Girls.—If it be conceded that there is need of physical exercise for boys, what must be said of the need of it for girls? Observe the young girls of cities and towns as they pass to and from school. Instead of the high chests, plump arms, comely figures, and graceful and handsome carriage, what do we constantly see? Flat chests, angular and warped shoulders, scrawny necks, slender arms and waists, and a weak and tired gait. Scarcely one in a dozen is thoroughly erect, whether walking, standing, or sitting. There is no elasticity in their steps, and a fresh, blooming complexion is so rare as to attract attention.

The girls of the most favored families often show the poorest physical development. The tyranny of fashion begins at a very early period in life. The quality and fit of the clothing worn by girls from ten to thirteen years of age prevent them from engaging in active, hearty play. The nurse or governess finds a large share of her duty in repressing that superabundance of spirits which should belong to every healthy girl.

As the years increase, the studies multiply, and by the time she is ready to leave school and assume the duties of life, we find a brain-weary, nerve-exhausted, pale creature, with no physical development, no power of endurance, and no ambition to undertake her share of life's duties.

When the importance of physical culture is as well understood as it should be, there will be a course of training for pupils of all ages in every girls' school in the land. In the larger cities and towns, provision is now made for physical instruction in many of the High Schools, but in the middle and lower grades, where the foundation should be laid and the work begun, the subject is almost wholly neglected. Bad habits of sitting, standing, walking, and breathing are acquired, and many forms of structural weakness developed which not only unfit the mind for the best work, but which later either become ineradicably fixed, or require much time and labor to correct. The schoolgirl, if systematically trained from early childhood, would show similar fruits of drill, and would develop into a shapely, graceful, well rounded, healthy girl, and would escape much of the weakness and suffering so common to women.

Herbert Spencer, speaking of the effects of the intellectual cramming system upon the women in England, and of the disadvantages of neglecting physical culture, says: "On women the effects of this forcing system are, if possible, even more injurious than on men. Being in a great measure debarred from those vigorous and enjoyable exercises of the body by which boys mitigate the evils of excessive study, girls feel these evils in their full intensity. Mothers, anxious to make their daughters attractive, could scarcely choose a course more fatal than this which sacrifices the body to the mind. Either they disregard the tastes of the opposite sex, or else their conception of those tastes is erroneous. Men care comparatively little for erudition in women, but very much for physical beauty and good nature and sound sense."

Symmetrical Development of Women.—The common argument of the busy housewife, when urged to take exercise, is, that she gets enough of it in the course of her daily duties, and even more than enough, for she finds herself thoroughly exhausted by the necessary labors of the day. The argument is not so convincing as it might seem. Doubtless, some of her muscles are overtaxed. They lack the support which the idle muscles should give. A few minutes, several times a day, devoted to strengthening the unused muscles, would not only afford relaxation to the tired ones, but, by developing the general strength, would prevent fatigue on the part of those most used.

Amount of Exercise Necessary for Women.—The amount of daily exercise necessary to regain health and develop strength depends upon the woman's present condition. If she is weak, generally, the exercise for the first fortnight, while comprehensive enough to bring all the muscles into play, must be light and easy. As strength is gained, the exercise may be gradually increased. As soon as a sufficient basis of vigor is reached, the essential thing to do is to adapt the exercise mainly to the weaker muscles so that they may catch up.

The right arm is usually stronger than the left. For the first month or two, give the left arm nearly all the exercise, gradually increasing the amount until it is able to do its share equally with the right. If the chest is small and the muscles of the back are weak, select the exercise specially suited to the case. The greatest care must be taken not to overdo the matter. For two or three weeks, only the mildest form of exercise should be employed, but the drill must be persistently kept up and gradually increased in difficulty. If the instruction or counsel of a specialist can be obtained, it would be well to secure it. If not, the wide range of valuable exercises given in this volume will be helpful in selecting and practicing those best adapted to the individual case.

If her work is of a sedentary or confining kind, there is the greater need of special exercise. Such work demands a strong constitution, and many break down under it annually. If long hours in shop, or store, or office are required of her, still it will be possible to find some time for exercise. Five or ten minutes may be secured upon rising in the morning. Clad in a loose robe, throw up the window and engage in vigorous, free hand gymnastics to expand the chest, increase the respiration, stimulate the circulation, and afford a healthy exhilaration to the muscles. After breakfast, walk to the place of business, or, if the distance be too great, walk part of the way. At noon, from five to ten minutes can again be secured for a breath of fresh air and a little exercise. A brisk walk with a cheerful companion will banish the dull routine of labor, and impart new energy for the duties of the afternoon. Even without the companion, the freer respiration induced by the walk, together with change of scene and thought, will prove beneficial.

In the middle of the forenoon, and again in the afternoon, three minutes can be found in which to stretch the cramped muscles and relieve the weary back. Stand erect, and with hands on hips and shoulders thrown back, take four or five full inhalations. Throw the hands over the head, and stretch them towards the ceiling, at the same time raise the heels, stand on the toes for a few seconds, and repeat about five times. This simple exercise, which need not occupy more than three minutes, will impart new energy, and result in the accomplishment of more work.

If an evening walk cannot be had every day, at least three or four might be enjoyed in a week, and would be productive of untold benefit. Let the motion be energetic and the step elastic. The distance should be moderate at first, and gradually increased. To this should be added five to ten minutes' exercise for the arms and chest before retiring.

This simple programme, involving no expense for apparatus, and requiring only so much time as even the busiest of men or women can find, will, in a short time, if persistently pursued, improve the digestion, stimulate the circulation, banish sleeplessness, transform dullness into cheerfulness, prevent weakness, impart tone and vigor to the nervous as well as to the muscular system, and contribute largely to the prolongation of a life of happiness and success.

Women of Leisure.—The daughters of wealthy or well-to-do parents and the wives of prosperous husbands should be the healthiest and happiest of women. Between graduation day and the wedding day, the young woman is frequently a lady of leisure. At least, she can usually control her time, and secure an hour or more each day for those healthful recreations which will fortify her against the various forms of physical weakness that are so common among women.

Out-Door Exercises.—Being free to enjoy the many out-door exercises, she should spend much time in the open air, making such choice of games and recreations as will bring into play the largest number of muscles, and afford the best all-round development, having in view, not only the securing of health and strength, but also the acquisition of grace and beauty.

Gymnasiums.—If a capable instructor and a gymnasium are at hand, she should avail herself of both. Supplementing her out-door sports with these, she will, in a year's time, unless already afflicted with some organic ailment or serious constitutional weakness, be so healthy, strong, and well developed, as to give promise of a long life, free from the infirmities that so commonly affect the sex.

Occupations of Men.—The vital statistics, preserved by many progressive states and communities, afford opportunity for fruitful study and comparison. Of all occupations, that of the farmer or gardener conduces most to health and long life. His independent manner of living, the pure country air he breathes, the abundant sunshine he enjoys, the plain, wholesome food he eats, his restful, quiet sleep, and his freedom from the demands of fashionable life, all combine to give him health. But this occupation, in itself, probably brings into play a larger number of muscles than any other single employment.

We cannot all be farmers, but whatever our occupation, there is much we can do to promote health, and to secure that happiness which is so largely dependent thereon. Many occupations afford exercise to a limited number of muscles, and those engaged therein should strive to find their recreation in the exercise of other muscles, so as to promote a well-rounded development. Persons who labor in-doors, and especially those who are confined to close workshops, stores, and schoolrooms, should have out-door recreation, with pure air and sunshine.

Unbalanced Bodies.—Many lines of mechanical trade afford sufficient exercise to keep the workman in fairly good health, yet few, if any, give a symmetrical physical development. The blacksmith and stone mason usually have strong right hands and arms, while the left are less fully developed. Nine-tenths of all machinists are right-handed. In nearly all mechanical industries, the right arm and the back have the larger share of the work, while the chest and leg muscles and the left arm are neglected.

Indifference.—Some workmen are so indifferent to physical symmetry that they are not willing to do anything to avert the one-sidedness resulting from their daily toil, even when convinced that a slight effort would correct the fault. The argument of increased health and vigor, and prolonged life, scarcely appeals to them.

Few persons are ambidextrous. Many more might use the hands with equal skill, if they would. Even so simple an operation as putting on a coat, using the wrong arm first, or buttoning a vest with the other hand, is awkward for most persons, and quite difficult to many. The best time to begin is in childhood, but, even if, when first learning the use of tools, the left hand is often made to do the work of the right, the exchange will prove restful to the overworked hand, and the symmetrical development of both sides of the body will be preserved.

A skillful teacher of music, in a private school near Philadelphia, suffered a partial paralysis of his right arm, which prevented its use for several years. This necessitated the increased use of the left hand, which resulted in its increased skill and power. Several years later, he removed to the South, where the warmer climate gradually restored the use of the right arm. By this time, the left hand had become almost as skillful as the right had been, and the severe affliction proved to be a blessing in disguise.

Brain Workers.—The brain workers are usually men of sedentary habits. To no class is exercise so important. Without it, some part of the human machinery is almost certain to get out of order. It may be the stomach or lungs, the liver or kidneys, the head, or eyes, or throat. There is a lack of perfect action of one or more of the parts, a clogging of the organs of digestion, or circulation, or respiration. This physical clogging at once affects the mental work, dulling the thinking powers, and often rendering their efforts futile, and making the complete cessation of labor necessary.

Headaches and indigestion are among the first ailments resulting from a lack of exercise. A brisk walk of twenty minutes or half an hour is often sufficient to dispel a headache. The exercise flushes the parts most actively engaged, and so depletes the brain. The same exercise stimulates the action of the lungs, makes better blood, quickens the activity of the other organs, and so tones up the whole man.

A young man, whose Christian zeal prompted him to devote all his spare time to religious work, ignoring the demands of health, broke down, and after a prolonged sickness, followed by a slow and tedious convalescence, was heard to remark, "Well, this experience has taught me one thing; the Lord has no use for a sick man." Had this young man taken a reasonable amount of exercise, he would have lost no time from his business, would have accomplished vastly more work for the religious organizations to which he belonged, and would have saved himself the pain, suffering, and expense of his sickness.

If the man who has eight or ten hours of busy brain work in-doors daily, and who, when his duties are ended, has no heart for physical exercise, would, every hour or two, turn aside from his work, and take even two minutes' vigorous exercise, in his office or in the adjoining hallway, he would return to his labor with brain considerably refreshed, and at the close of the day, he would enter upon his half hour's walk with spirit and alacrity, and welcome his sleep at the end of the day.

Business Men.—Who does not know, among his business acquaintances, men whose faces show that they are continually overworked? They have no time for systematic physical exercise, but go dragging through their duties as well as their low physical condition and tired brains will permit. The noonday lunch is bolted, or is omitted entirely, for want of time.

Dr. S. Weir Mitchell, a specialist in nervous disorders, speaks of the numerous instances of nervous exhaustion among merchants and manufacturers. He says: "My note books seem to show that manufacturers and certain classes of railway officials are the most liable to suffer from neural exhaustion. Next to these come merchants in general, brokers, etc.; then, less frequently, clergymen; still less often, lawyers; and, more rarely, doctors; while distressing cases are apt to occur among the over-schooled young of both sexes."

Few business or professional men do anything to secure and preserve health and strength, and they go through life far less efficient and useful than they might be.

Pre-eminent business success can be achieved only by turning over to subordinates the numerous details which occupy so much time, and which any trustworthy and experienced secretary or assistant might do. By this arrangement, time would be saved for necessary recreation and rest, thus keeping the physical systems of the employers and managers in the best possible condition, and securing to the mind that alertness and vigor which the sharp competition of the times demands.

Professional Men.—Looking over a list of eminent divines, it is surprising how many of them were men of rugged frames and sturdy physique. It required a man with the physical vigor of Luther to declare he would attend the Diet of Worms "though the devils there were as numerous as the tiles on the houses." How much of the success of Spurgeon, and

Beecher, and Dr. John Hall may be fairly ascribed to their splendid outfit of vital organs, and to the glowing health which each enjoyed. Nor were Phillips Brooks, and Joseph Cook, and Dwight L. Moody lacking in these physical qualities which count for so much in influencing the minds and hearts of men. These knew nothing of "blue Mondays" or "ministers' sore throat," and needed not to be sent abroad by their congregations, every summer or two, in order to recruit their health, and keep them up to their work.

By virtue of his profession and because of its onerous and responsible duties, no one stands more in need of robust health than the physician. Called from his bed at all hours of the night, brought in daily contact with disease, and that often of a contagious character, the largest demands are made upon his vital forces. He is expected, not only to dispense the necessary medicines, but also to carry comfort and cheer to the bedside of the sick. The very countenance of a healthy, cheerful physician acts like a medicine.

The country practitioner who rides or drives long distances, over rough roads, and who often attends to his horse himself, needs but little further exercise, and that little should be applied to the least-used muscles, in order to preserve a well-rounded development. The city physician, whose coachman relieves him of the exercise of driving and of the care of the horses, will find a half hour daily, with pulley-weights, clubs, or dumb-bells, and an occasional visit to a gymnasium conducive to his best physical condition. As a dentist should himself have the best of teeth, the doctor also should enjoy the most robust health.

And what of the legal profession? Rufus Choate inherited a strong, healthy body, but took so little care of it, that, towards the close of his life, he was accustomed to say of himself that "latterly he had worn out his constitution, and was living on the by-laws." He died at fifty-five, while his contemporary, Daniel Webster, who appreciated the importance of keeping his body well toned-up, and who, with fishing rod in hand, found recreation among the streams of his native State, preserved his robust physique and imperial bearing to the allotted three score and ten. Lord Brougham, as a boy, was the swiftest runner in his neighborhood. His physical strength and endurance were such that upon one occasion he spoke in Parliament seven days consecutively. He kept up his activity to the end of his life, and died at the age of eighty-nine.

President Eliot, of Harvard College, who has enjoyed exceptional opportunities for observing the effects of exercise upon young men, says: "A singular notion prevails, especially in the country, that it is the feeble, sickly children who should be sent to school and college, since they are apparently unfit for hard work. The fact that, in the history of literature, a few cases can be pointed out in which genius was lodged in a weak or diseased body, is sometimes adduced in support of the strange proposition that physical vigor is not necessary for professional men. But all experience contradicts these notions. To attain success and length of service in any of the learned professions, a vigorous body is well-nigh essential. A busy lawyer, editor, minister, physician, or teacher has need of greater physical endurance than a farmer, trader, manufacturer, or mechanic. All professional biography teaches that to win lasting distinction in sedentary, in-door occupations, which task the brain and the nervous system, extraordinary toughness of body must accompany extraordinary mental powers."

Heredity.—In the matter of bodily health and vigor, the sins of the parents are visited upon the children. What narrow-mindedness the father displays, therefore, in devoting himself so assiduously to business as to neglect his health, and to entail upon his sons and daughters such a low standard of vitality as to impair their usefulness in life, and to deprive them of the power to enjoy, as they should, the inheritance he hopes to leave them.

Exercise for the Stout, the Thin, and the Old.—It may seem somewhat paradoxical that the same means that are employed to increase flesh and weight should also be recommended to reduce obesity. There is a difference, however, between superfluous fat and solid, healthy, active muscle.

The Stout.—It is a well known fact that persons of moderate weight, in preparing for some unusual or extraordinary test of strength, reduce their flesh and toughen their muscles by a course of severe training. It is not an uncommon thing for college crews to reduce their weights, by a month's training, twelve pounds per man. A prize fighter will often come down thirty or forty pounds in preparing for a contest. An instance is cited of a student, who, after carefully weighing himself, sat down to a fifty-five pound rowing-weight, pulled forty-five full strokes a minute for twenty minutes, then, with the same clothing as before, weighed himself, and found he had lost one pound.

Many men, and women, too, if persuaded that there was, at hand, a convenient and comparatively easy method of ridding themselves of their burden of flesh, would doubtless avail themselves of it. The following well authenticated cases may be suggestive and helpful. A young lady, inclined to fleshiness, by vigorous horseback riding, reduced her weight twenty-five pounds in one year. A policeman, whose weight was three hundred and fifteen pounds, took a position as stoker on a war vessel. The exercise, coupled with the free perspiration induced by labor in the heated quarters, lowered his weight to one hundred and eighty-four pounds. A man in middle life, whose occupation was a sedentary one, and whose weight, over three hundred pounds, was a source of great discomfort, resolved to try what exercise would do. Being much engrossed through the day, he began by taking long, brisk walks in the evening. Soon he was able to cover five miles at a fairly good pace. Whatever the state of the weather, and however tired he might be with the day's exacting duties, he suffered nothing to interfere with his evening walk. He gradually increased the pace and the distance, and, with little or no change in his diet, in five months he had taken off ninety pounds. He says that he often perspired so freely that, in cold weather, small icicles were formed on the ends of his hair. Free perspiration is a necessary element in the rapid reduction of flesh. The fat-producing foods should be avoided as far as possible.

While exercise is one of the best means of reducing superfluous fat, there is no class of persons more loath to take exercise than the obese. The reasons are largely physiological. The greater weight is a burden to carry. The muscular tissues have in part changed to fat, and are therefore less able to do their work. The action of the lungs and the heart is interfered with by the pressure of the fat, and the individual quickly becomes exhausted and short of breath. There is the greater demand, therefore, on the part of those who incline to obesity, to exercise with determined persistency and regularity, in order to reduce their weight. Exercises involving quickness of movement, and a degree of mental activity, are the best.

The Thin.—The old proverb says: "It is a poor rule that will not work both ways." Judged by this standard, the rule of exercise must be a good one, for the instances of lean arms and legs filled out, and of scrawny necks and hollow shoulders made round and plump by exercise, outnumber the other ten to one.

Many lean persons, impressed with the apparent discomfort and inconvenience of obesity, are content with their slender measure of flesh. This is especially true of men, who, as a rule, have less regard for beauty of form than those of the other sex. They overlook the fact that the man whose bony structure is well overlaid with thick layers of healthy muscular tissue is able not only to accomplish more work, but to stand greater exposure and endure more hardships than the lean man. His stronger, heavier muscles will not only carry his greater weight with less effort, but his larger body will possess a momentum that the other man does not have.

In the severe training preceding the inter-collegiate boat races, while the over fleshy lose their superfluous fat, the thin gain as rapidly in weight. Many lean people whose occupations are of a physical nature do too much, daily, in proportion to their strength. Mind and body are kept in such a constant state of activity that their energies become exhausted. If such persons will take an occasional rest through the day, when it is possible so to do, and will add an hour or more to the period of sleep, their weight will soon begin to increase. Then, by special exercises aimed at the weak points, and persistently sustained, the gain in weight will be that of solid, healthy, muscular tissue, which will not only fill out their leanness, but will give them power to do more work with less fatigue.

A short rest after meals, with the practice of deep abdominal breathing, begun, if need be, as a special drill, but ultimately established as a habit, will go far toward improving the digestion and converting the food into good, healthy blood, so indispensable to the growth of every part of the human body.

Exercises for Gouty and Rheumatic Persons.—Gout and other uric acid conditions, whether hereditary or acquired, frequently yield to systematic physical exercises. These conditions are generally the result of indigestion or overfeeding. By exercise, more oxygen is brought into the circulation of the blood, and the chemical process is promoted. By free perspiration, the action of the skin is stimulated, and the work of the kidneys is lightened. In the case of those afflicted with gout, special care is needed for a time. A mild form of exercise should be employed at first, and gradually increased. A free perspiration should be induced daily, followed by a bath and vigorous rubbing.

Exercises for the Dyspeptic.—If the system has become much weakened by dyspepsia or indigestion, begin with mild forms of exercise—walking, bicycling, golf, and other out-door sports. For a lack of tone of the abdominal muscles, swimming in warm weather is found useful. The in-door tank is not quite so good as the stream or surf. If the liver is chiefly at fault, horseback riding is a capital remedy. Gradually introduce more vigorous exercises. Daily bathing and rubbing must not be neglected.

Exercises for the Development of Special Muscles.—Few persons, even among those who have given considerable attention to physical culture and have spent much time in a gymnasium, could, if asked, tell what special forms of exercise were best calculated to fill out a hollow shoulder or flat chest, or strengthen weak loins or back. The following suggestions will therefore prove helpful.

The different muscles of the human body are so closely interwoven that it is impossible to exercise one without, at the same time, giving exercise to another lying contiguous to or co-operating with it.

The Chest.—While it is important that all the muscles of the body should be exercised, those that are most closely allied to the vital functions of respiration, circulation, and digestion claim the first consideration.

Breathing Exercises.—For the purpose of chest expansion, nothing can take the place of regular breathing exercises. While respiration is an involuntary act, yet the manner is, to some extent, subject to the control of the will. There are three commonly recognized forms of breathing—the clavicular, the costal, and the abdominal. These are not wholly independent, but overlap each other.

Clavicular Breathing.—Place the palms of the hands on the chest, with the tip of the middle finger resting on the clavicle, or collar bone. Inhale slowly, directing the breath toward the upper chest. Hold the breath a few seconds, then exhale slowly. Repeat ten to fifty times.

Costal Breathing.—This is a fuller and better form of breathing than the clavicular. The lower ribs are more flexible than the upper, and, supplemented by the action of the intercostal muscles, admit of freer movement of the lungs. Press the hands against the sides. Inhale through the nose, and inflate the lungs to the fullest. Hold the breath as long as convenient. Exhale forcibly through the open mouth. Repeat five to ten times. Repeat, exhaling slowly through the nostrils. Repeat, exhaling through a small glass or other tube, with an aperture about the size of an ordinary knitting needle. While the lungs are inflated, strike the chest gently with closed hands. This will drive the air into the remotest cells. With the lungs filled, and the arms akimbo, bend the body at the waist, forwards, backwards, and from side to side, and return to erect position before exhaling.

Abdominal Breathing.—This is the best method of breathing, and should be cultivated by all. Singers and speakers find in this the fulcrum of their vocal power. The contraction and expansion of the diaphragm, that wonderful muscular partition, which separates the thoracic from the abdominal cavity, affords the largest and freest movement of the lungs, and, by its pressure upon the viscera, repeated with every breath, it aids greatly in promoting digestion. Many persons, especially women, do not employ abdominal breathing to the extent they should. Some, indeed, hardly know its meaning.

Upon retiring at night, remove all constricting bands about the waist, lie upon the back, and rest the hands upon the abdomen. Direct the breath so as to raise the hands. Fill the lungs full as possible, and hold the breath for several seconds. Exhale, letting the hands fall with the outgoing breath.

Take two or three ordinary breaths, then repeat, drawing in the breath slowly through the nostrils, lock in the breath for a few seconds, and exhale slowly as before. A better position of the body would probably be secured by folding a comfortable, spreading it upon the floor, and lying flat upon the back. Heavy pillows and yielding bed-springs crook the body, and often prevent the best results. The abdominal movement, in breathing, is not quite so apparent when standing or sitting, but if the exercise be taken as frequently as possible, with the mind directed to the freest diaphragmatic movement, the habit of full, deep, abdominal breathing, with its numerous attendant advantages, will soon become established.

Chest Muscles.—Not only should the lung cavity be enlarged by breathing exercises, and by any physical exercise that stimulates respiration, as steady and protracted running, but the front chest should be well covered by the pectoral muscles. With the arms at right angles to the body, and with head thrown back, so as to face the ceiling, raise and lower the dumb-bells from twelve to eighteen inches. As strength increases, increase the weight of the bells and the number of lifts. Swinging with the hands upon the horizontal bar is another good exercise. The "dips" exercise, elsewhere referred to, is also good for the pectorals, but must not be attempted until after strength has been gained by lighter exercises. The relation of the biceps and triceps to the pectoral muscles is so close that any exercise for the former will be helpful to the latter.

Respiratory Exercise, No. 1.—With arms at sides and elbows stiff, raise the hands as high as possible above the head. Rise upon the toes at the same time, so as to give the body the longest possible upward reach. Inhale slowly through the nostrils while the arms ascend, and hold the breath a moment or two, then exhale, lower the arms, and rest back upon the heels. Repeat ten to twenty times. It is needless to say that in the in-door exercises, and especially in the breathing exercises and those which stimulate respiration, the room should be well ventilated. The head and neck should be held erect, except where a different position is required.

Respiratory Exercise, No. 2.—Lie flat upon the floor, face downward, hands folded upon the back. Inflate the lungs and lift the head and shoulders as high as possible, giving out the breath slowly. Repeat several times, and as strength increases, oftener.

Abdominal Exercise, No. 1.—Several good exercises for the abdominal muscles are here given, which can be taken upon rising in the morning and upon retiring at night. With just enough clothing to keep the body from chilling, lie flat on the back upon a folded comfortable spread upon the floor. Without bending the knee, raise the foot toward the ceiling as far as possible, then the other foot, so alternating ten times or oftener. Next raise both feet together. While these movements should be brisk, the limbs should not be allowed to drop back upon the floor, but the muscles should be kept tense. Next, from the vertical position of the leg, bend the knee and press it closely upon the abdomen for a moment, then restore to the vertical position and lower to the floor. Alternate the limbs as before, then take them together.

By means of a loop, or other simple arrangement, to keep the feet from rising, lift the head and trunk to a vertical position by contracting the abdominal muscles. This is a severe exercise, and should not be attempted by those who have any special abdominal weakness. The strain may be relieved, however, by propping the head and shoulders with pillows, so as to make, with the lower limbs, an angle of about forty-five degrees. Gradually, as the abdominal muscles increase in strength, take out one pillow after another, until able to raise the body from the horizontal position. The latter exercise may be still further graduated by first resting the arms at the sides; next cross them on the chest, and then clasp the hands behind the neck before lifting the trunk. In gymnasiums it is not an uncommon thing to see a person with well developed abdominal muscles lift another person lying prostrate across his chest, and weighing anywhere from one hundred and fifty to two hundred pounds, by the sheer force of these muscles.

Abdominal Exercise, No. 2.—Sit on a bench or stool, and with feet under a couch, or hooked into a strap fastened to the base-board of the room, with arms folded upon the chest, bend forward and backward, as far as possible, without strain. Repeat ten to twenty times. After a few weeks, increase the bend.

Abdominal, Side, and Back Muscles.—Stand erect with hands on hips. Keep head, neck, and legs rigid, and lungs well filled. Bend slowly backward and forward several times. Bend from side to side. With feet firmly planted, bend forward, and revolve the head and trunk to the right, back, left, front, and assume an erect position. Bend forward again, and reverse the order of movement. Repeat several times. Next, stand erect, with hands firmly planted on hips, and twist the body from the waist upward, first to the right as far as possible, then to the left, and repeat ten to twenty times.

The Loins.—The muscles in the small of the back, running up and down on each side of the spine, come into play in many forms of manual labor, and should therefore possess strength and endurance. Working with the shovel, or fork, or bar, or saw, or any exercise requiring a stooping posture, brings them into action. Several of the exercises recommended for the abdominal muscles will prove of advantage here. Raising dumb-bells above the head, first with the left hand, then with the right, then with both, beginning with bells weighing a pound or two, and each month, with daily practice, adding a pound to the weight until it reaches about one-twentieth the weight of the person, will bring the desired results. Running or rapid walking, with the body erect, will prove helpful. Hopping straight ahead for from five to ten steps on one foot, then on the other, and thus alternating for from twenty to one hundred steps, or more, will soon beget strength, and give a firm, steady carriage.

The Back.—The muscles of the back, above the waist line, participate in nearly all the movements recommended for the chest, shoulders, and upper arm, and do not require special exercises.

The Shoulders.—To round out hollow shoulders and put muscle on the upper back, stand erect, with light dumb-bells, arms hanging at the sides. Without bending the elbow, keep the arms parallel, and carry the bells backward and forward as far as possible. Hold for a few moments, and slowly return to the sides. Repeat five to ten times. As strength increases, gradually add to the weight of the bells and the number of lifts, also endeavor to carry the arms a trifle higher. For developing the muscles of the shoulders, back, and wrist, few exercises are better than light Indian-clubs.

For the outside of the shoulder, bring the arms to the horizontal, elbows rigid, and move the bells up and down through a space of twenty inches. Repeat five to ten times. Carry to the front and repeat. A few weeks of daily practice should show noticeable results, and a year of persistent drill will produce a shapely shoulder, and make it unnecessary for the tailor to pad the coat in order to make it fit.

The Neck.—The muscles of the neck may best be developed by the use of a strong rubber strap, about two feet long. Attach one end to the door frame, about the height of the head when standing, and fasten the other end to a band which loosely encircles the head. The front, back, and sides of the neck may all be strengthened and filled out with firm, shapely muscles, by changing the position of the body for each change of exercise desired. Keep the head firm to resist the pull of the strap. Increase the length of the movement and the strength of the pull, as the muscles grow strong to bear it.

The Upper Arm.—The biceps is the large front muscle of the upper arm. It bends the arm and brings the hand toward the shoulder. A large biceps is the envy of many young men who regard it as the criterion of physical strength, and who often develop it out of all proportion to the rest of the body. It is, however, an important muscle, and should receive due consideration. Most persons will find that one arm or one leg or one side is weaker than the other. Give to the weaker member much the larger practice until the equilibrium is restored, then exercise them equally.

With dumb-bells, flat-irons, window-weights, or other objects in hand, slowly bend the arm until the hand almost touches the shoulder, then slowly lower to position. Repeat ten to twenty times. Gradually increase the weight and the number of lifts. If pulley-weights are used, stand so that the outstretched hand barely reaches the handle of the rope. With palms upward, draw the hand toward the shoulder. Slowly relax and repeat.

When away from home, and having no access to anything that may serve as apparatus, in this, as in many exercises, one arm may serve as lever and the other as weight. With the right hand, grasp firmly the wrist of the left. Press down vigorously with the left, but use enough force to overcome the resistance, and with the right raise it to the shoulder. After several repetitions, reverse the hands.

Some persons ignore the use of all apparatus, preferring what is known as free gymnastics. This extreme is greatly to be preferred to that of using heavy, and often dangerous, appliances. In many exercises, the weight of the body or its parts affords sufficient resistance to develop the muscles. In other cases, the imagination supplies the want of resistance, and, by due concentration of will, making one set of muscles pull against another, the muscles may be given as much work as though actual weight were present. To children and young persons, light and suitable apparatus will furnish added stimulus and interest.

Climbing a ladder or rope, hand over hand, or lifting the body so that the chin may touch a horizontal bar overhead, are exercises better suited to later stages of biceps development. To be able to lift the body to the bar with one hand, three to five times, should satisfy any reasonable ambition.

The triceps are the back and inside muscles of the upper arm, and contribute much to the shapeliness as well as usefulness of that member. Instead of stopping at the shoulder, as in the biceps exercises, push the dumb-bells high overhead. Any exercise of pushing with the arms is of advantage. Stand back about two feet from the door, grasp the sides of the frame a trifle higher than the shoulders, and, rising on the toes, with head erect, thrust the body forward. Press back until the body again assumes an erect attitude, and repeat ten to twenty times.

The Forearm.—Many of the exercises for the upper arm and shoulder have a very direct bearing upon the forearm. Most of the mechanical occupations requiring the use of axe, saw, plane, hammer, shovel, plow, or any tool or instrument requiring a firm grasp of the hand, develop these muscles. The lifting of a heavy weight suspended from a bar or handle, to be grasped by the hands, produces speedy results, but must not be attempted until the muscles of the back, abdomen, and shoulders have had preparatory training.

The Hand.—In the exercises already described, the hand and wrist will have received much valuable training for strength of hold or grip. A firm grasp of the oar, the bat, the bar, or the heavy hammer is apt to leave the hand with an ungainly hook when at rest. Counteract by pressing the fingers forcibly against the wall, or, in lifting the body from the floor in the triceps exercise, use only the fingers and thumbs instead of the palm. The wrists may be exercised by twisting the dumb-bells at arm's length in front, at the side, and overhead.

If the fingers are weak, train them individually, beginning with the weakest. Always bring up the weakest part first, and aim to secure and preserve proper symmetry throughout. The pulley-weights are excellent for the purpose. Attach a small strap to the handle, and begin with such weight as will afford exercise but will not overtax the finger. Pull ten to thirty times. In the absence of pulley-weights, lifting, by a strap, a box of sand or bricks or any weight that can be gradually increased will serve the purpose. Drive a stout nail or screw into the upper part of the door frame. Throw the strap over the nail, and lift the body, first using two fingers, then one. Trained gymnasts lift the entire weight of the body several times by the little finger alone.

The Thigh.—Fast walking, running, jumping, hopping, skating, and dancing are all good for developing the front of the thigh. More rapid development will be secured by standing erect, slowly bending the knees as if about to sit in a chair. Hold the body in that position for several moments, and slowly rise to an erect posture. Repeat ten to twenty times. After two weeks of daily practice, lower the body until the back part of the thigh rests on the calf. Rise slowly as before. Repeat ten to twenty times. After a month, increase the weight by carrying dumb-bells, bricks, or other objects in the hands. When this has become easy, hold one foot front or back, and have the other leg do the lifting.

The under part of the thigh, in the ordinary occupations and recreations of life, does not get as much exercise as the front muscles. A slovenly, shambling gait is characterized by a feebleness of this muscle, while a strong, elastic step is accompanied by a well developed under thigh. With knees unbent, stoop over and try to touch the floor with the fingers, making five or ten thrusts before assuming an erect attitude. Walking or jumping up and down on a plank elevated at an angle of forty-five or fifty degrees with the floor, with the toes toward the higher end, is a good exercise for the calves and the under thigh. Stand on one foot, weight the other, and swing it backward and forward as high as possible.

The Calf.—Climbing up hill, running on the toes, hopping long distances on one foot-any one of them, if persistently followed, will, in a short time, result in strengthening the calf and increasing its size. Professor Maclaren declares that in four months of Alpine climbing his calves increased from sixteen inches to seventeen and one-quarter, and his thighs from twenty-three and one-half inches to twenty-five.

Another exercise, very simple, has been found productive of great good. Stand erect, chest out, shoulders down, knees stiff, feet slightly apart, toes turned outward. Raise the heels as high as possible, throwing the weight of the body upon the toes. Repeat at the rate of fifty to seventy times a minute. One minute's work will prove sufficient for the exercise. Increase to two, three, or four minutes a day for a month. A gentleman, approaching middle life, who was not satisfied with a calf that girthed fourteen and one-quarter inches, in four months, by this exercise, added another inch. He devoted fifteen minutes to it, morning and evening, and after a time carried a twelve pound weight in each hand.

Pulley-Weight.—The uses of the pulley-weight are so numerous and so varied that it constitutes almost a complete gymnasium in itself. One of its prime advantages is, that by gradually multiplying the number of weights, it adapts itself nicely to the increasing strength of the individual, and to the varying powers of the different members of the family. It reaches directly every muscle of the hand, wrist, arm, shoulder, chest, abdomen, back, and neck. By the use of an extra pulley near the floor, necessitating a longer rope, excellent drill of the leg muscles is afforded. By sitting on the floor, the latter arrangement is converted into a rowing machine, affording exercise for the arms, back, and legs.

Dumb-Bells.—These are less expensive but scarcely less valuable than the pulley-weight in the scope and variety of the exercises they afford. They may be of wood or iron, and should not be heavy. For the average person, one and one-half pounds, each, is a good weight. For children, one pound is sufficient.

A Home-Made Gymnasium.—By a home-made gymnasium is meant the use of such appliances as the ordinary home will furnish, or as a person, with a little mechanical skill, can supply.

Chair Exercises.—A light chair, grasped firmly by the outer upright supports of the back, with the two hands, and swung vigorously around the head ten to twenty times, first in one direction, then in the other, will afford one of the best simple exercises known. It brings into play the muscles of the hands, arms, legs, and many parts of the body, and if repeated at short intervals will not only increase the respiration and stimulate the circulation, but will also start the perspiration. The intervals should be occupied with exercises that bring into play other muscles, as rising on the toes, stretching the legs, breathing exercises, etc.

Another valuable chair exercise consists in placing two chairs, front to front or side to side, with a space between them of about six inches more than the width of the body. Place the hands flat on the chairs, then slip the feet back, and with the toes resting on the floor and the limbs and body rigid, lower and raise the body several times. For deepening the chest and strengthening the arms and shoulders, this will be found an excellent exercise.

Unless the chair feet are spread, care must be taken to place the hands well within the edge of the seat, to prevent the chairs from tipping over. One chair may be used instead of two, by grasping the sides of the seat firmly and bringing the chest nearly or quite to the front of the seat.

Door-Jamb Exercise, No. 1.—A light form of chest and arm exercise may be had by grasping the side jambs of a door-frame, about as high as the shoulders, and planting the feet a short distance back. Keep the lower limbs and trunk rigid, the head thrown well back, and thrust the body backward and forward from ten to twenty times.

Door-Jamb Exercise, No. 2.—For those having weak chests and weak arms there is no better exercise than that known as the "dips," for which the parallel bars of the regular gymnasium are largely used. An excellent substitute for the bars may be made by boring a hole about two inches in diameter into each side of the door-frame, about waist high, and fitting to each hole a strong wooden handle or peg. These should project into the doorway with a space of eighteen to twenty inches between their inner ends in which to stand. The exercise consists in placing the hands on the pegs, and slowly raising and lowering the body a number of times by the muscles of the arms alone. At first, some assistance from the toes may be necessary. Soon the arms will be able to do the work alone. Beginning with five lifts, the number may be gradually increased to fifty. It is understood that the pegs may be removed when not in use.

If the disfigurement of the door-frame between two rooms, or room and hallway, is a serious objection, the jambs of a roomy closet door may be used, in which case the closing of the door shuts the holes from sight. Two high tables, or a foot rail of a bed and a table, or box placed firmly upon two chairs—in short, any two pieces that will afford a lift of the body, such as that described, will serve the purpose nearly as well.

Door-Jamb Exercise, No. 3.—By fastening two cleats or supports on the inner faces of the door-frame, with a niche or slot in each, to support a horizontal bar, extending across the doorway near the top, just within reach, a simple but very valuable piece of apparatus is ready for use. For strengthening the fingers and the grasp of the hands, as in swinging back and forth by the arms, and in developing certain arm, back, and abdominal muscles, as in lifting the body so as to touch the chin to the bar, few exercises are better. The latter was a favorite exercise of William Cullen Bryant, and one to which he attached much value. It is attended with some danger, however, and should not be attempted without preparatory drill. The sides of the bar, at the ends where it enters the cleats, should be slightly flattened, so as not to turn with the swinging motion of the body. Two or three sets of cleats may be used, adapting the height to different members of the family.

REST

Its Necessity.—Rest is as necessary as exercise. We cannot be active continually. Repose must succeed labor. Alfred the Great is credited with the recommendation that each day be divided into three parts, eight hours for labor, eight hours for recreation, and eight hours for sleep.

Change of Employment.—A change of occupation affords rest. The wood chopper finds relief from his ax by using his saw. A different set of muscles is brought into play. Persons might often save themselves from excessive fatigue by the adoption of this principle. When physical labor is made to alternate with mental activity, the sense of rest is more apparent.

Sleep.—The best form of rest is found in sleep. All voluntary activity then ceases. Even the involuntary processes of circulation and respiration seem to share in the general restfulness, for during sleep their action is more tardy, and, as a result, the temperature of the body is somewhat lower. More covering is needed during sleep than during the waking hours.

While the body is in action, the process of pulling down predominates, but during sleep nutrition goes on, the wasted tissues are built up, and we rise refreshed and prepared for the new day's duties.

Amount of Sleep.—All persons do not require the same amount of sleep. It is said that Frederick the Great slept only five hours each night. Napoleon Bonaparte could pass days with only a few hours' rest. Persons whose labors are mental require more sleep than those who work with their hands.

The average person in good health requires eight hours' sleep. Children, invalids, and the aged need more. Those who take less should make a careful study of themselves to ascertain whether they get all the refreshment of mind and body that they need. If sleep is insufficient, it will show itself sooner or later in general lassitude and weakness. The imperative demands of Nature are shown in the recorded instances of sailors on war vessels falling asleep on the gun-deck while their ships were in action, of soldiers falling asleep on the march, and even persons falling asleep on the rack in the intervals of their torture.

Position While Sleeping.—An active, healthy child will sleep well in almost any position, but a nervous, wakeful person, who is obliged night after night to woo sleep, must study what conditions are most conducive to its attainment.

Most persons sleep best on the right side. In this position the stomach is easily emptied, and the liver does not press upon the heart and stomach. Those affected with heart trouble will experience less oppression and distress in this position than by sleeping on either the back or on the left side.

The Pillow.—A high pillow, especially if firm and unyielding, cramps the neck and interferes with respiration and circulation. Some writers upon health advocate the use of no pillow, but most persons, either from habit or for more substantial reasons, find a pillow of moderate size to be of advantage.

The Mattress.—The old-time bed-ticking filled with clean oats straw, thoroughly shaken up each day, and renewed once or twice a year, made a thoroughly comfortable and wholesome bed. In these modern days, hair, cotton, felt, and corn husk are the substances most commonly employed. A good mattress is neither too soft nor too hard, but yields to the exterior bony processes of the body without engulfing the sleeper. Feathers, once very widely used, are now generally condemned by physicians and sanitarians.

Rest During the Day.—Almost everyone has experienced the invigorating influence of an after-dinner nap during the long days of summer. Many persons would accomplish more work by taking a rest of ten or fifteen minutes once or twice a day at all seasons of the year. To women in poor health, and to those who are overworked, this suggestion has special application. It not only rests the tired muscles but it soothes the nerves, and serves as a most refreshing tonic. Instead of being a loss of time, it will prove to be time saved. More actual work, both of hands and brain, will be accomplished, and with less expenditure of vital force. Dr. William Pepper accomplished an immense amount of work with but very little sleep. It was not unusual for him, when sorely in need of rest, to break off in the midst of his work, lie down and immediately go to sleep, and after five or ten minutes wake up refreshed.

DWELLINGS

Site.—In the selection of a home, due regard should be had to the site. High ground is more healthful than that which is low; a loose, dry, sandy, or gravelly soil is better than one that is wet and clayey. Made ground, as a rule, is unhealthful, as it is usually low to begin with, and is commonly filled up with earth which contains more or less organic matter.

Soil.—The interstices of the soil are occupied by air, or water, or both. The impurities of the soil mingle with the ground air, and render it unfit for breathing. When this ground air is forced above the surface by an influx of water or by the pressure of the heavier air above, much danger lurks in the surface atmosphere. Damp cellars and basements should be avoided, and the upper rooms of the house selected for living and sleeping rooms. Careful scientific investigation has established a close connection between cholera, typhoid fever, malarial fevers, and the rise and fall of the water in the soil.

Dr. Henry I. Bowditch, of Boston, some years ago, formulated these two propositions:

First, A residence in or near a damp soil, whether that dampness be inherent in the soil itself or caused by percolation from adjacent ponds, rivers, meadows, or springy soils, is one of the principal causes of consumption in Massachusetts, probably in New England, and possibly in other portions of the globe.

Second, Consumption can be checked in its career, and possibly—nay, probably—prevented in some instances by attention to this law.

The truth of these propositions was, later, corroborated by Dr. William Pepper, of Philadelphia, and by Dr. Buchanan, of England. It is even suspected by certain physicians that some of the prevalent diseases among horses and cattle are due to dampness of the soil.

Drainage of the Soil.—In view of the above facts, the importance of draining wet soil is obvious. A noted scientist states that ground in which the water is sixteen or more feet below the surface is uniformly healthy; when it is less than five feet, it is always unhealthy; and that a fluctuating level, especially if the changes are sudden, is very unhealthy. Certain trees and plants, such as the eucalyptus and the sun-flower, whose roots absorb a prodigious quantity of water which is given off through the leaves, are useful in drying wet soils.

The close connection between various forms of disease and the condition of the soil has many times been pointed out. Some years ago, the British government instituted an examination of the effects of drainage in twenty-four towns. While the results indicate a general diminution of the death-rate, the deaths from consumption show the greatest reduction. All forms of malarial disease, fever and ague, neuralgia, influenza, dysentery and other diseases of the bowels are also greatly reduced by draining wet soils.

Duty of the Householder.—It should be the first duty of every householder to secure perfect means for conveying beyond the walls of his domicile everything of a dangerous character that is generated within it, and to secure his home against the entrance of foul air, impure water, or unusual dampness. While the responsibilities of the dweller in the city are shared by the city officials, in that the city supplies the water and provides the sewer to carry off the waste from the kitchen, lavatory, and toilet, yet the householder needs to see that absolute cleanliness is observed, that the pipes are regularly flushed, and the traps kept in good working order, that no decomposing substances are permitted to give off their poisonous gases in cellar, alley, or yard, and that the cellar and foundation walls are free from excessive moisture. The dweller in the country has the additional responsibility of securing and preserving a pure water supply, and of providing proper means for the disposal of the waste of the household.

Dry Cellars.—The floor of the cellar should be covered with an impervious concrete. The foundation walls, especially if built of soft stone, should be furnished with a course of hydraulic cement or other impervious material, and the inside surface thoroughly coated with the same. Where there is a heater or furnace in the cellar, the evils of dampness are somewhat reduced during the winter months while the fires are kept going. If the soil is wet or springy, a drain of ordinary field tile of small size should be laid all around the inside of the cellar walls, and, together with the rest of the cellar floor, should be covered with concrete.

Kitchen Drains.—In many country houses this is the only drain, and it is often the source of incalculable mischief, due in most cases to sheer carelessness. The drain pipe need not be large—four inches in diameter is sufficient—but it must be kept free of obstruction, so that the waste from the kitchen may pass off rapidly, and no part of it be suffered to lodge, to decompose, and to send its death-distilling gases back to the kitchen, and thence through the other rooms of the house. Not only should the outlet of the kitchen drain be kept away from the well or cistern, but no part of the drain pipe should come within twenty feet of it. The best of pipes and joints, unless frequently renewed, are apt to break, and a very small aperture leading from the drain pipe into the source of supply of drinking water may endanger not only the single household but the entire community. A well of infected water in London, spoken of as "the Broad Street pump," and famous in the annals of epidemics, is known to have caused the death of over five hundred people in a single week.

Drinking Water.—So large an amount of sickness has been directly traced to an impure water supply that too much emphasis cannot be placed upon the need of proper precaution. Not only should the ground about the top of the well be banked to throw off surface water, but the upper wall of the well, for a distance of five or six feet from the surface of the ground, should be laid in cement, and the space between the wall and the ground filled in with wet clay well puddled around the curbing.

If a gravel seam or loose porous rock lies between the well and the cess-pool, even when these are a considerable distance apart, there is absolute danger, unless the receptacle for the waste products of the household be made thoroughly water-tight. Without this precaution, the well may be safe for a few months or even a year or more, but sooner or later the foul fecal matter will reach the source of water supply, carrying with it disease and death. No odor or taste may mark the inflow of polluted matter. Some of the most dangerous well-waters are sparkling in appearance and refreshing to the taste.

Sewage.—Few subjects relating to health are of greater importance than the proper disposal of the refuse and waste matter of the household. Even if free from the specific germs of disease, the organic matters contained in sewage give rise to noxious emanations, which, when inhaled, lower the tone of the system and render it an easy prey to disease.

Dangers of the Soil Pipe.—It is chiefly through the soil pipe that cess-pool and sewer gas finds its way into the house. The return of these foul emanations is often caused by the force of their own expansion and sometimes by the pressure of the sewer air behind them. The water-traps afford but a slight barrier to their progress. Every drain pipe leading to cess-pool or sewer should be connected with a ventilating shaft which will carry the foul vapors above the roof of the house, and as far away from the windows as possible.

The Medical Officer for Edinburgh, in a recent report, declared that wherever water-closets had been introduced, in the course of one year there were double the number of deaths from typhoid and scarlet-fever, and that any epidemic fever occurring in these houses assumed a character of malignant mortality.

Disinfectants.—Chemical disinfectants are used by many good housewives, and are helpful, but they cannot be wholly relied upon. Cleanliness, ventilation, and dryness are the natural disinfectants. Artificial disinfectants can no more be substituted for them than perfumes can be made to take the place of soap and water.

Sewer Gas.—This poisonous gas is known chiefly by its effect. It frequently passes the water-traps and enters our sleeping and living rooms, there to do its fatal work. The alternate floods of hot and cold water open the joints of iron pipes, and allow the gas to escape. Leaden gas pipes decay and become perforated, with the same result. Dr. Fergus, in his pamphlet "The Sewage Question," says: "For some years I have insisted on a careful examination of the soil pipes wherever I have cases of typhoid or diphtheria, and in every case where I could get this carefully carried out I have detected perforated pipes, or have found sewer air getting into the houses in some other way. In many cases the plumbers have declared pipes to be all right, which turned out to be very defective when uncovered."

Water-Traps.—These are not so effective in preventing the escape of sewer gas as they are considered to be. Experiments with glass tubes shaped and arranged just as the ordinary water-traps in sinks and closets are arranged have shown that the light gases pass through by the top of the bend, and the heavy gases by the bottom. A rush of wind up the mouth of a sewer, or a heavy dash of rain which fills the sewer and reduces the air space, so increases the pressure of the gas within the sewer and soil pipe that the ordinary water-traps are not able to resist it.

Water-traps that are not used for a time become death-traps. The water soon evaporates, and affords an unobstructed channel for the conveyance of foul gases from cess-pool or sewer to the rooms of the house. Houses that are vacated for the summer, and that are without tenants for a time, should be thoroughly cleaned and ventilated, and have all pipes and drains flushed with water before being occupied.

Size, Flow, and Fall of Drain Pipes.—The efficiency of a drain or sewer depends upon its capacity, its slope or incline, and the velocity of its flow. If the amount of water flowing is proportionate to the size of the conduit, sewers of different sizes give the same velocity at different inclinations. A ten-foot sewer with a fall of two feet per mile, a five-foot sewer with a fall of four feet per mile, a two-foot sewer with a fall of ten feet per mile, and a one-foot sewer with a fall of twenty feet per mile will have the same velocity provided they are filled in proportion to their capacity. The ten-foot sewer will require one hundred times as much sewage as will the one-foot sewer. If it has less, the velocity of its stream will be correspondingly diminished. It is especially important, therefore, that the size of the conduit be adapted to the volume of the stream, as well as to the slope or inclination.

An experienced engineer gives a velocity of three feet per second as the least that should be allowed for the outlet drain of a house. To secure this flow a four-inch drain should have a minimum inclination of one inch in ninety-two; a six-inch drain, one in one hundred and thirty-seven; a nine-inch drain, one in two hundred and six; and to attain the above velocity of three feet per second at these inclinations they must run not less than half full. The great purpose of all modern sewage systems is to carry off all waste matters before they have time to decompose.

Joints of Drain Pipes.—These should be made so smooth within as not to impede the flow of sewage, nor become obstructed by catching thread, strings, hair, and other floating substances. They should be so tight as absolutely to prevent any leakage of either fluid or gaseous matter, and render impossible the entrance of the small filaments of the roots of trees growing along their course. They should be supported on solid pillars of brick or stone, and not spiked to cellar walls where a slight settling will force the joints and cause a leak. They should be so firmly supported at every point that after the joints have been cemented no possible change of direction or slope of pipe can occur. Any such change is sure to work disaster.

Sewer Ventilation.—No sewer is safe that does not have a free current of air passing through it. Motion and aeration are the safeguards against infection. Sewers should be constructed so as to secure a constant flow, with no sharp angles or short turns to impede its progress, and with frequent vents leading to the surface of the street. Thus diluted, the sewer gas becomes harmless, the pressure in the conduits is relieved, and the danger of the gas forcing its way through the water-traps into the living and sleeping rooms of our homes is avoided.

Location of Closet.—The water closet should be so placed as to have an exterior window, by means of which it may be fully ventilated. Under no circumstances should the closet open directly into the bedroom. When entered from the hallway or landing, the conditions may be improved by cutting off half of the space as a vestibule or outer apartment, thus preventing any foul odors from reaching the sleeping rooms. For reasons of convenience as well as of health the bath-room and lavatory should be separate from the water closet.

Disposal of Garbage.—In cities, the public authorities collect and dispose of the solid waste of the kitchen. In the country, and wherever chickens, cows, or pigs are kept, these waste substances may be utilized. Some private families burn them. Where this cannot be done they should be removed from the dwelling far enough to prevent their decomposition from giving rise to any unpleasant or unwholesome odors. No compost heap should be maintained within one hundred yards of a dwelling.

Dry Earth Closet.—This system of disposing of the waste matter of the household is not so well known in the United States as it is in England, where it has been in successful use for many years. The best apparatus is that invented by Rev. Henry Moule, an English clergyman.

The following claims are made for it, and they are supported by the best authorities:

1. It furnishes a comfortable closet on any floor of the house, and it may be supplied with earth and cleaned of its deposits by the servants without the intervention or knowledge of any member of the household.

2. It furnishes a portable commode in any dressing-room, bedroom, or closet, the care of which is no more disagreeable than that of an ordinary fireplace.

3. It affords appliances for the use of immovable invalids which entirely remove the distressing accompaniments of their care.

4. It provides for the complete and effectual removal of all liquid waste of sleeping-rooms and kitchen.

5. It completely suppresses the odors which, despite the comfort and elegance of modern living, still hang about cesspools and privy-vaults, and attend the removal of their contents.

The expense is trifling as compared with that of water sewerage. The care and attention needed is somewhat greater, and this probably accounts for the limited use of the system in this country. In country houses, and in small towns and villages where the facilities of a system of public sewerage are not to be had, it would seem that the advantages of the earth-closet system would commend it to general favor.

The earth-closet is a mechanical contrivance attached to the ordinary seat, for measuring out and discharging into the vault or pan below a sufficient quantity of sifted dry earth to entirely cover the solid ordure and to absorb the urine. The earth is discharged by an ordinary chain or wire-pull, similar to that used in the water-closet. The vault or pan beneath the seat is so arranged that the accumulation may be readily removed. In a small family once in two or three weeks is often enough to empty the pan or drawer unless it is small. The entire apparatus need not cover more than two feet square by three feet high.

It is estimated that our present wasteful method of disposing of the night-soil occasions an annual money loss to the country of over $100,000,000. When the economic value of human excreta becomes as well known in the United States as it is in China and Japan we will cease to cast it into the sea.

A Truthful Picture.—Any one who has lived among or mingled much with people in the country and in hamlets and villages will recognize the truthfulness of the following picture as presented by George E. Waring, Jr., in "How to Drain a House." He says:

"Let us see what chance a woman living in the country has to escape the direst evils that 'delicate health' has in store for its victims. The privy stands perhaps at the bottom of the garden, fifty yards from the house, approached by a walk bordered by long grass, which is always wet except during the sunny part of the day, overhung by shrubbery and vines, which are often dripping with wet. In winter, snow-drifts block the way, and during rain there is no shelter from any side. The house itself is fearfully cold, if not drifted half-full with snow or flooded with rain.

"A woman who is comfortably housed during stormy weather will, if it is possible, postpone for days together the dreadful necessity for exposure that such conditions imply. If the walk is exposed to a neighboring workshop window, the visit will probably be put off until dark. In either case, no amount of reasoning will convince a woman that it is her duty, for the sake of preventing troubles of which she is yet ignorant, to expose herself to the danger, the discomfort, and the annoyance that regularity under such circumstances implies.

"I pass over now the barbarous foulness and the stifling odor of the privy-vault. It is only as an unavoidable evil that these have been tolerated; but I cannot too strongly urge attention to the point taken above, and insist on the fact that every consideration of humanity, and of the welfare not only of your own families, but of the whole community, demands a speedy reform of this abuse. * * * I make no apology for calling the attention of women themselves to this important matter, believing that they will universally concede that, however much of elegance and comfort may surround them in the appointments of their homes, their mode of life is neither decent, civilized, nor safe, unless they are provided with the conveniences that the water-closet and the earth-closet alone make possible."

Woman's Part in Sanitation.—Some years ago, Dr. B. W. Richardson, then president of the British Medical Association, said: "I want strongly to enforce that it is the women on whom full sanitary light requires to fall. Health in the home is health everywhere; elsewhere it has no abiding place. I have been brought indeed by experience to the conclusion that the whole future progress of the sanitary movement rests for permanent and executive support on the women of the country. When, as a physician, I enter a house where there is a contagious disease, I am, of course, primarily impressed by the type of the disease, and the age, strength, and condition of the sick person. From the observations made on these points, I form a judgment of the possible course and termination of the disease; and, at one time, I should have thought such observations sufficient. A glance at the appointments and arrangements and management of the house is now necessary to make perfect the judgment. The men of the house come and go; know little of the ins and outs of anything domestic; are guided by what they are told; and are practically of no assistance whatever. The women are conversant with every nook of the dwelling, from basement to roof; and on their knowledge, wisdom, and skill, the physician rests his hopes."

Materials of the Dwelling.—No material is so dry and healthful as wood. Where the dangers of fire preclude the use of this material, as in close and compact cities and towns, and where brick and stone must be employed, such houses may, with very slight additional expense, be rendered comparatively dry. Ordinary bricks absorb a great deal of moisture, and carry dampness from cellar to attic. Soft building stone is nearly as bad. The use of a double course of vitrified brick on a thick layer of the best cement just above the foundation wall, or ground line, will prevent the dampness of the soil from being carried up through the walls. The outside dampness from rains and sleet may also be corrected by the use of thick studding against the walls on the inside to support the plastering. This leaves an inch or two of space between the outer wall and the plastering, through which the air can circulate, and thus preserve the inner walls of the dwelling from dampness.

Lighting.—The Italians have a proverb, "When you let the sunshine in you drive the doctor out." A house should be constructed so as to admit an abundance of light. Architects, and builders, too, often undervalue the health-giving properties of sunshine, or sacrifice them to other considerations. Even the mistress of the house, whose first thought should be the health of herself and that of her children, frequently shuts out the sunshine to save her carpets and furniture. It is better to have the roses on the children's cheeks than on the carpets.

Trees should not be planted so close to a house as to obstruct the free ingress of light and air. If the walls are damp, the tree's shade will help to preserve the dampness. Numerous instances are recorded of the deaths of persons clearly traced to the damp walls, moss-covered roofs, and general unhealthfulness arising from the close proximity of dense trees which overhung the dwelling and shut out the sunlight. When the sad truth was at last discovered, and the trees were removed, the houses which, before, were seldom free from sickness and sorrow, became wholesome and cheerful.

Warming.—The subjects of warmth and ventilation are so closely related that they will necessarily overlap in their treatment. In point of importance probably no two subjects have a larger bearing upon health. No scheme has yet been devised by which satisfactory means of heating and ventilation are combined with money-saving. For purposes of ventilation, the old-time open hearth was without a rival. But while the faces of our grandparents were roasted, successive chills chased up their backs. In these days of scarcity of fuel, the open hearth is the rich man's luxury.

Most houses throughout the country are still warmed by stoves. In cities and towns, dwelling houses are generally warmed by the hot-air furnaces, while many of the larger establishments—stores, offices, hotels, banks, apartment houses—are supplied with steam heat.

An important consideration in all cases of hot-air heating is that the air be taken from the outside through a conduit instead of using the air from the cellar, as is too frequently done. In some cities and suburban towns, pure air is brought into the cellar through a conduit where it passes through a box in which it is heated by steam pipes, the steam being brought from a central plant which supplies several hundred houses. The air when heated passes through flues to the several rooms of the dwelling, and is turned on and off by registers in the usual way. This system avoids all dirt of coal and ashes, and all care of fires, and is much to be commended.

Uniform Temperature.—In all schemes for the warming of houses, it is important to keep the entire building at a uniform, comfortable temperature. In dwellings, the halls and living rooms should be so evenly warmed that no sensation of chilliness is felt in passing from one room into another. This, in itself, costs much fuel, and when there is added the further cost of heating the fresh air which is necessary to supply the place of that which has become vitiated by use, the truth of the proposition that suitable heating and ventilation are costly becomes apparent.

Those who live in warm, close, ill-ventilated rooms are much more subject to colds from exposure to draughts and cold air than those who dwell in a pure atmosphere of moderate temperature. This being the case, persons should not accustom themselves to a higher temperature than is barely necessary for comfort. Some persons are most comfortable with a room temperature in winter of 68° or 69° Fahrenheit. Others require a temperature of 70° or 71°. Invalids, infants, and old persons, whose vitality is low, require a higher temperature than those in the full vigor of life.

Ventilation.—The importance of breathing pure air was fully discussed in a previous chapter. The best methods of securing it will be considered here.

Air, when heated, becomes lighter and rises. Cool air, when it enters a warm room, sinks to the bottom. The cooler and purer air of a room is, therefore, always found nearest the floor. Although the carbonic acid given out by the lungs is heavier than an equal quantity of atmospheric air, yet, by the operation of the law of diffusion, it commingles with the other gases, and is found in greatest quantity near the ceiling. Doors and windows are the means commonly employed for ventilation; transoms and special ventilating flues are used to some extent.

Where large numbers of people are congregated together for several hours at a time, as in churches, theatres, and public halls, proper ventilation becomes a matter of extreme importance. If, in such cases, doors and windows alone are depended upon, the results are never satisfactory. Those nearest the windows are made uncomfortable by the chilling drafts, while the persons in the middle of the room experience very little relief from the stifling atmosphere. In the construction of such buildings suitable provision should be made in floor, side-wall, and ceiling for an ample supply of pure air, without a conscious current or other annoyance to the audience. In school houses, where children are confined for long periods, and where their physical growth and mental activity demand the purest air, neglect of proper means of ventilation on the part of school directors and trustees is little short of criminal.

In the home the subject of ventilation during the day time is a simple matter. The frequent opening of outer doors and of inner doors, with the occasional lowering of the upper sash of the window, will furnish an abundant supply of pure air.

The ventilation of the sleeping room is not always so simple, especially where privacy demands the bolting of the chamber door. The diminished vitality of the individual during sleep requires that there shall be no draft over his bed. If there be but a single window, place the bed so as to escape the draft. Lower the upper sash about two inches. If there be two sleepers in the room lower it three inches. Raise the lower sash an inch or two. This gives three air spaces, top, bottom, and in the middle where the two sashes overlap. A thin board placed on edge in the window ledge, and fitting inside the window strip, will throw the current of air upward, and when the wind is strong, will prevent a draft. A transom over the door stimulates a gentle current of air, and is of great advantage. In some families, where privacy permits, the door is left slightly ajar at night. This, with a slight opening of an outer window, will secure ample ventilation.

Air Currents.—A current of two feet per second is scarcely perceptible; of three feet is quite noticeable; of five feet is a positive draft. In introducing fresh air into a room the current should nowhere exceed two feet per second at the point of entrance.

Individual Requirements of Air.—Each adult person requires three thousand cubic feet of air per hour. This will demand an opening or place of entrance equal to twenty-four square inches, and an equal amount of space for the foul air to escape. An opening four by six inches will give much more air than one twelve by two inches by reason of the smaller friction upon the sides. Ventilation through a single pipe or aperture is more effective than that through several apertures of equal aggregate area.

Stairs.—Many persons, especially women, who, as a rule, do more stair climbing than men, find it very exhausting. Some stairs are easier to mount than others. In the construction of stairways, architects and builders should reduce the labor to the minimum. The wants of a certain invalid necessitated a constant going up and down stairs. The successive nurses were wont to remark, "I never saw, before, such an easy flight of stairs." The exact measurements of this stairway are: seven and one-eighth inches rise; eleven and one-half inches depth, or space from the front edge to the back part of each step. There is a landing near the middle. A landing gives the climber an opportunity to get a full breath, and greatly reduces the effort of mounting.

www.ingramcontent.com/pod-product-compliance
Lightning Source LLC
Chambersburg PA
CBHW080523030426
42337CB00023B/4615